LOW RESIDUE COOKBOOK

A COMPREHENSIVE DIET GUIDE AND COOKBOOK WITH OVER 130 LOW FIBER DAIRY FREE AND GLUTEN FREE RECIPES FOR PEOPLE WITH CROHN'S DISEASE, ULCERATIVE COLITIS, AND DIVERTICULITIS

MONET MANBACCI, PH.D.

(Edition-1)

Copyright © 2020 by Monet Manbacci.

All Right Reserved.

Healthview Publishers

Disclaimer Notice

No part of this publication may be reproduced, distributed, or transmitted in any form or by any means, including photocopying, recording, or other electronic or mechanical methods, or by any information storage and retrieval system without the prior written permission of the publisher, except in the case of very brief quotations embodied in critical reviews and certain other noncommercial uses permitted by copyright law.

Please, consider that the information in this book is only for educational purposes. No warranties of any kind are implied or declared in this book. Readers acknowledge that the author of this book is not engaged in the rendering of medical, legal, financial, or professional advice. Hence, consult a licensed professional before applying any hints or techniques outlined in this book. By reading this notice, the readers agree that the author of this book is not responsible for any direct or indirect losses that are incurred because of the use of the information contained in this book, including but not limited to inaccuracies, omissions, and errors.

This book has been published by the Healthview Publishers. All rights reserved.

Table of Contents

Disclaimer Notice 2
Introduction 10
Chapter 1: Low Fiber and Low Residue Diets 13
    Low Fiber Diet 13
    Liquid Diet 13
    Low Residue Diet 14
Chapter 2. Comprehensive List of Foods to Avoid & to Eat 16
    Fruits 17
    Vegetables 19
    Herbs 22
    Spices 24
    Oils 25
    Animal Proteins 26
    Seafood 28
    Whole Grains 29
    Refined Grains 30
    Gluten-Free Flour Options 31
    Nuts 32
    Seeds 33
    Legumes 34
    Sweeteners 35
    Dairy Products 36
    Lactose-Free Yogurt Products 37
    Butter 38
    Lactose-Free Milk Products 39
    Cheeses 39
    Sauces, Dips, and Gravies 41

Ready Foods (In General) 43

Chapter 3. How to Cook in Low Residue Diet 47

    Cooking Styles/Methods 47

    Food Ingredients 48

        Fruits and Vegetables 48

        Rice, Noodle and Pasta 49

        Meat and Poultry 50

        Seafood 52

        Grains 52

        Soy, Eggs, and Firm Tofu 54

        Dairy Products 54

        Spices and Herbs 55

        Cheese 56

        Oils 57

        Sauce, Gravy, Salad Dressings 57

    Drinks 59

    Meals 59

        Breakfast 59

        Soups 60

        Salads 60

        Snacks 61

        Desserts 62

        Side Dishes 63

Chapter 4. Food Preparation & Meal Planning 64

    Eating Habits 64

    Grocery Shopping 65

    Cooking Tools 67

    Kitchen preparation 68

    Meal Planning 68

Chapter 5. Low Residue Diet Cooking Recipes 70

   Breakfasts 70

      Gluten-Free Fluffy Pancake 70

      Banana and Apple Pancakes 71

      Eggs, Salmon, and Avocado 73

      Baked Apple 74

      Pear Oatmeal Bars 75

      Avocado & Egg Breakfast Toast 77

      Smoothie Bowl 79

      Zucchini Bread Oatmeal 80

      Breakfast fruit salad 81

      Banana Split Oatmeal 83

      Egg Tacos with Avocado 84

      Crispy Hash Brown with Egg 85

      Grilled Almond Butter Honey Banana Sandwich 87

      Avocado-Cheese Bagel 88

      Apple Cinnamon Oatmeal 89

   Appetizers 91

      Turkey Potpie Soup 91

      Potato-Ginger Miso Soup 93

      Parsnip/Carrot Potato Soup 94

      Pumpkin Soup 96

      Stracciatella Soup 97

      Ham and Potato Soup 99

      Butternut Squash Soup 101

      Chicken Noodle Soup 102

      Creamy Chicken Soup 104

      Seafood Chowder Soup 106

      Barley/Oatmeal Soup 107

- Homemade Vegetable Broth 109
- Homemade Beef Broth 111
- Russian Chicken Soup 113
- Baba Ghanoush 114
- Salmon Bruschetta 116
- Guacamole-Like Appetizer 117
- Homemade Lebanese Hummus 119
- Crab Dip with Wonton Chips 121
- Shrimp Salad 123
- Zucchini Salad (Spiralized) 124
- Olivier Salad (Chicken, Potato & Egg salad) 126
- Apple-Pear Salad with A Special Vinaigrette 127
- Beet, Carrot & Apple Salad 129
- Butter Lettuce Salad with Honey Vinaigrette 130
- Carrot-Avocado Salad 131
- Classic Tuna Pasta Salad 133
- Salmon Ceviche 134
- Honey Chicken Salad 136

Main Courses 138
- Mediterranean Chicken - Zucchini Stew 138
- Lactose-Free Chicken Fettuccine Alfredo 140
- Chicken with Mashed Potatoes 142
- Chicken Stroganoff 144
- Chicken Kebab 146
- Roasted Chicken with Pomegranate Sauce 148
- Puffy Chicken 150
- Chicken Scaloppini 152
- Chicken Pizza 153
- Turkey Zucchini Noodles 155

Zucchini Egg Dish 156

Potato Cutlet 158

Ginger Sticky Pork 159

German Pork Schnitzel 161

Baked Apple Pork 163

Balsamic-Peach Pork 164

Honey-Turmeric Pork 166

Grilled Lean Beef Kebab 168

Hungarian Goulash 170

Tomato Free Spaghetti Bolognese 172

Lamb/Beef Liver stew 174

Grilled Honey Salmon 175

Oven-based Salmon and Potato 177

Lemon Steamed Halibut with White Rice 179

Thunfisch Pizza 181

Avocado Tuna Pita 182

Trout with Orange 183

Chicken and Shrimp Teriyaki 185

Lemon Shrimp with White Rice 187

Honey Prawn Linguine 188

Desserts 190

Pear Cake Sundaes 190

Apple-Ginger Sundaes 192

Banana Lemon Trifle 193

Warm Apple Crumble 195

Apple Quesadillas 196

Middle-Eastern Rice Pudding 198

Gluten-Free Apple Pie 199

Pumpkin Pie 201

Fruit Dessert..203

Avocado Pear Popsicle..204

Lemon Sorbet..206

Ingredients..206

Mango Ice Cream..207

Sweet potato pie...209

White Panna Cotta..210

Cocktails and Shakes..212

Banana Milkshake...212

Cooler Drink...213

Mango-Banana Smoothie..214

Ginger Cool Drink...215

Avocado Smoothie..216

Banana-Cinnamon Smoothie..217

Peach-Mango-Banana Smoothie...218

Peach-Ginger Smoothie..219

Pomegranate-Angelica Smoothie..220

Apple-Ginger Smoothie..222

Bloody Red Drink!..223

Papaya-Mango Smoothie..224

Cantaloupe Smoothie...225

Cantaloupe-Mix Smoothie..226

Applesauce-Avocado Smoothie..227

Pina Colada Smoothie..228

Snacks..230

Diced Fruits..230

Plain Yogurt with Poached Fruits...230

Poached Fruit Compote..230

Applesauce...232

Homemade Applesauce 232
Avocado Dip 233
Homemade Hummus 235
Tofu 237
Avocado Tofu Toast 237
Almond Butter Sandwich 238
Gluten-Free Muffins 239
Cheese Sticks 241
Avocado Tuna Toast 242
Rice Crackers 243
Gluten-Free Rice Cracker 243
Ginger Biscuits 245
Gluten-Free Ginger Biscuits 245
Zucchini Chips 247
Healthy Potato Chips 248

Drinks 249
Recommended Hot Beverages 250
Recommended Cold Beverages 253

Chapter 6. Bi-weekly Cooking Plan 256
Cooking Plan for Remission Periods: 256
Cooking Plan for Flare-Up Periods 259
Biweekly Cooking Plan for IBD patients – Blank 262

Last Words 265

One Last Thing 267

About The Author 268

Other Books By Healthview Publishers: 269

Introduction

The Low Residue Diet mostly follows by people with inflammation bowel disease (IBD), such as Crohns's disease or Ulcerative Colitis or other gastrointestinal disorders such as diverticulitis. In such patients, fiber is not digested or absorbed well in the gastrointestinal system, causing abdominal pain, bloating, gas, diarrhea, and nausea in some cases.

If you or your loved one has been diagnosed with any of the diseases that needs you or your loved one to follow the low residue diet, you already know how hard such disease could be and how tough it can be managed. Research studies have found that many issues come from the followings:

- Not knowing much about the intolerance
- Self-treatment
- Ignoring signs and symptoms
- Not knowing about triggering foods to avoid
- Mismanagement of the disorder
- Not following the doctor's orders correctly or completely

One of the best ways to manage your symptoms, and have a healthier life, is to follow a "Low Residue" diet or a "Low Fiber" diet, with the help of a comprehensive diet guide and cookbook.

This book gives the readers valuable information about healthy nutritional choices, foods to eat or to avoid, food preparation, meal planning, and how to create biweekly cooking plans based on low-residue diet. It primarily provide readers with necessary nutritional information about the condition and then, guide readers on their cooking and dietary plans. This book is recommended to the groups below:

1. You need to follow the low residue diet and want to know how to manage your diet, how to cook varieties of foods, and how to balance your meals using effective meal plans.
2. You have a family member and want to know how to prepare low residue meals or make meal plans.
3. You recently realized that you need to follow a low residue diet and do not know how to cook for yourself
4. Your loved one newly diagnosed with a gastrointestinal disorder and needs to follow a low fiber or a low residue diet.

If you have recently diagnosed or if your loved one have recently diagnosed with IBD, IBS, or any other gastrointestinal disorders, this book is an excellent source for you to take initial necessary dietary steps, learn how to cook varieties of low residue and low fiber foods, how to manage your disorder, how to do meal planning and learn about diet tips.

In addition, following a bad diet can certainly cause issues when it comes to choosing what you eat and drink. Not only does the condition cause digestive tract irritation and uncomfortable symptoms, but long-term consequences may include malnutrition. To make matters more complicated, your dietary habits may worsen symptoms. Eating and avoiding certain foods explained in this book can help prevent symptom flares. That is why one of the chapters of this book focuses on food preparation and meal planning.

Comprehensive lists of foods to avoid and foods to eat are presented in this book as well. The book then fully covers how to cook with low fiber foods following by more than 120 low residue diet cooking recipes. This chapter covers various types of recipes for breakfast, appetizers, soups, salads, snacks, main courses, desserts, and drinks. Each recipe starts with a brief explanation, preparation time, cooking time, total time, ingredients, instructions, cooking tips, Low residue diet-related tips, and nutrition facts.

The nutrition facts of the recipes in this book have been analyzed by "Verywell fit" Recipe Nutrition Calculator (Ref: https://www.verywellfit.com). Biweekly cooking plan samples are given to you in Chapter 6. The same chapter provides you with blank biweekly cooking plan tables for you to write your cooking plan and stick it to your fridge.

It has to be reminded that the recommendations, hints, and tips provided in this book have been gathered from various related research studies and references from different online/offline resources. These have been found useful by the author of this book, but it does not mean that all will work for you or for your loved one. It should be understood that any recommendations or tips in this book can only be followed only when you take responsibility for it. Be sure that you always talk to your doctor or dietician about the recipes, steps, or hints this book recommends to make sure that they are in line with your health condition.

Chapter 1: Low Fiber and Low Residue Diets

Low Fiber Diet

This diet is suitable for people who cannot have fiber for any reason. Doctors may recommend this diet to some of IBD or diverticulitis patients who had colon surgical procedures. The main idea is to avoid eating foods high in fiber. This diet is one of the diets that are great to follow if you have Crohn's, diverticulitis, or ulcerative colitis. Some foods to avoid in the low fiber diet are:

- Whole-grain foods such as brown rice & oat
- Anything whole wheat such as whole wheat pasta or bread
- Foods with seeds and nuts
- Corns and popcorns
- Berry fruits
- Lentils
- Granolas
- Dried fruits
- Foods that produce gas such as broccoli and cauliflower (not raw, not cooked)
- Raw fruits (exceptions: melon, banana, and skin removed peach)

Liquid Diet

Your doctor may ask you following a liquid diet in specific circumstances temporarily such as:

- Very hard flare-up

- After a surgical procedure
- Blockages or strictures in the large intestine

The main idea is to avoid solid foods for a while to give rest to the gut and quicken the healing process. You should be under the supervision of a doctor or a nutritionist to make sure that you receive the right nutrients while taking this diet. Here are some of the tips when you need to take a liquid diet:

- Consume bone broth, chicken broth, and vegetable broth a lot.
- Fresh fruit juices do not have much fiber. You can have fresh fruit juices from recommended fruits.
- It is recommended to purchase a juicer or a blender. Having a juicer is recommended as it can break down the fibers from your fruit/vegetable juices.
- Cook soups and then blend them with a blender.
- You can combine fruit juices with vegetable juices, as well.
- Drink plenty of water.
- Some patients can use Gatorade. Ask your doctor about it.
- Remove any pulp from the juices before drinking them.

Low Residue Diet

A low residue diet is another diet that can be asked to follow if you are an IBD patient or have other gastrointestinal disorders that cannot tolerate fiber well such as diverticulitis. This diet can add residue to the stool and can lessen diarrhea and abdominal pains and cramps, which is suitable for people with IBD who had surgeries in their large intestines.

Some of the foods to avoid in a low residue diet include, but not limited to:

- Nuts (including almond and coconut) and seeds
- Raw fruits such as berries
- Dried fruits
- Some fruit juices such as prune juice
- Raw and leafy vegetables
- Jams and marmalades
- Whole grains
- Pickles
- Strong seasonings such as pepper, chili, and garlic
- Legumes
- Popcorns and corns
- Hard to digest cheeses
- Fried and processed meats
- Fried eggs
- Fried foods and fried pastries

The recommended foods to allow and foods to avoid in this book are well-matched with a low-residue diet. Generally speaking, some diets recommended for IBD patients are high in proteins and high calorie, as some patients need to have a faster healing process. Your doctors may ask you to combine the low fiber diet with the low residue diet. In this case, you need to follow both diets at the same time. The next chapters of this book can help you write your diet plan based on the foods that you can well-tolerated during remission and flare-ups.

Chapter 2. Comprehensive List of Foods to Avoid & to Eat

This chapter provides comprehensive lists of foods to eat and foods to avoid for patients who wants to follow the low residue diet for flare-up and remission periods. To cover a variety of foods from "safe foods to eat," to "triggering foods to avoid," five different colors are defined as indicators as follows:

G	The food is safe to consume.
B	It is recommended to consume this food in moderation.
Y	Each patient needs to check this food to see if the food is tolerable or not.
O	It is recommended not to consume or limit taking this food.
R	Avoid consuming this food.

Different food categories are investigated, and the tips related to flare-up and remission periods are explained in this chapter.

As such, you can see one of these five colors in front of each food in food category lists, which can help you decide whether to go with that food item or not.

Remember, it does not mean that the foods highlighted in blue can be consumed without tolerance checking. It means that according to research studies, experiences of patients, or expert recommendations, they are more likely to be safe and non-triggering. Always test your tolerance regarding foods in blue color.

On the contrary, it does not mean that the foods highlighted in orange cannot be consumed. It means that according to research studies, experiences of patients, or expert recommendations, they are more likely to trigger. Always test your tolerance regarding foods in orange color, have your research and, if you decide to consume, have them in little amounts or use them in moderation. Table 2 to Table 22 present foods to eat and to avoid for flare-up and remission periods.

FRUITS

During Flares

1. In many cases (except not allowed fruits in red or orange), poached, skin and core-removed fruits can be well-tolerated.
2. Make sure you do not consume poached fruits, or compotes high in sugar during flares.
3. Do not forget to eat fruits in blue color in moderation during flares.
4. Check if a fruit increases diarrhea during flare-up periods or not. If yes, avoid using it.
5. Check if the fruit is high in fiber or not. Avoid consuming it if it has high insoluble fiber inside.
6. Check if the fruit is easy to digest or not. If it is hard to digest, avoid eating it during flares.
7. Check if the fruit can help dehydration or not. Consider other factors when you choose a fruit to eat during flares.
8. Check if a fruit has anti-inflammatory properties or not. Consider other factors when you chose a fruit to eat during flares.

9. Avoid fruits with non-removable seeds during flares such as berries.

During Remissions

1. You can consume fruits shown in green color during flare-ups, but it is recommended to peel off and remove cores of fruits during the remission period as well.
2. Most fruits can be well-tolerated during remission periods.
3. Remember to eat fruits in "blue color" in moderation.
4. Be aware of consuming orange or red fruits during remission periods.

Table 2. List of fruits to eat and to avoid

Fruits:	Flare-up	Remission
Apple	B	G
Apricots	O	B
Avocado	G	G
Banana Ripe	Y	G
Banana	B	G
Banana Unripe	B	G
Barberries	R	O
Blackberries	R	O
Blueberries	R	O
Cantaloupe	G	G
Carambola/Starfruit	G	G
Cherries	R	O
Clementine	O	G
Coconut	O	Y
Cranberries	O	B
Date	O	G
Dragonfruit	O	G
Durian	O	B
Feijoa	R	B
Figs	R	B
Goji berries	R	Y
Gooseberries	R	Y
Grapefruit	O	G
Grapes	O	Y

Guava	R	B
Honeydew Melon	G	G
Jackfruit	Y	G
Java-Plum	Y	G
Jujube Fruit	Y	G
Kiwifruit	O	B
Kumquat	O	G
Lemon	G	G
Lime	G	G
Longan	Y	G
Loquat	O	G
Lychee	Y	G
Mandarin	O	G
Mango	B	G
Mangosteen	Y	G
Mulberries	O	O
Nectarine	B	G
Olives	G	G
Orange	O	G
Papaya	G	G
Passion Fruit	O	B
Peaches	B	G
Pear	O	G
Persimmon	O	B
Pineapple	R	O
Plums	O	Y
Pomegranate	B	G
Prunes	R	O
Quince	O	B
Raisins	R	O
Raspberries	R	O
Rhubarb	R	O
Strawberries	R	O
Tamarind	B	G
Tangerine	O	G
Watermelon	G	G

VEGETABLES

During Flares

1. In many cases (except not allowed vegetables in red), boiled or steamed, skin-removed vegetables can be well-tolerated.
2. Make sure you do not stir fry vegetables during flare-up periods.
3. Eat vegetables in blue in moderation during flares.
4. Check if a vegetable increases diarrhea during flare-up periods. If yes, avoid eating it.
5. Check if a vegetable is high in insoluble fiber or not. If yes, avoid consuming it or boil it.
6. Check if a vegetable is easy to digest or not. If it is hard to digest, avoid eating it during flares.
7. Check if a vegetable has anti-inflammatory properties or not. Consider other factors when you chose a vegetable to eat during flares.

During Remissions

1. It is recommended to consume tolerable vegetables (raw or boiled) during the remission period.
2. Many vegetables can be well-tolerated during remission periods (highlighted in green).
3. Remember to eat vegetables in blue in moderation.
4. Try to consume vegetables with fiber, folic acid, vitamin A, C, E, and K, calcium, and other required nutrients for IBD patients.

Table 3. List of vegetables to eat and to avoid

Vegetables:	Flare-up	Remission (Raw)	Remission (Boiled)
Amaranth Leaves	R	O	Y
Alfalfa	R	O	Y
Arrowroot	R	O	Y
Artichoke	R	O	Y
Arugula	R	O	Y
Asparagus	R	Y	B
Bamboo Shoots	R	O	Y

Beans, Green	O	B	B
Beets	R	Y	B
Belgian Endive	R	O	Y
Bok Choy	R	O	Y
Broccoli	R	R	O
Brussel Sprouts	R	O	Y
Cabbage, Green	R	R	O
Cabbage, Red	R	R	O
Carrot	G	G	G
Cauliflower	R	R	O
Celery	Y	O	Y
Celery Root	R	O	Y
Chicory	R	O	Y
Collards	R	O	Y
Corn	R	R	R
Cucumber	B	B	G
Edamame	R	Y	B
Eggplant	O	Y	B
Fennel	R	O	Y
Ginger Root	B	B	G
Horseradish	R	O	Y
Jalapeño	R	R	O
Kale	R	O	Y
Kohlrabi	O	Y	B
Leeks	R	O	Y
Lettuce, Butter	B	B	G
Lettuce, Iceberg	R	O	O
Lettuce, Leaf	R	O	O
Lettuce, Romaine	R	O	O
Mushrooms	O	O	Y
Mustard	R	O	O
Okra	R	O	Y
Onion, Red	R	R	O
Onions	R	R	O
Parsnip	R	O	Y
Peas, Green	R	O	Y
Pepper, Green	R	O	O
Pepper, Red	B	O	O
Potato, Red	B	G	G
Potato, White	Y	B	G
Potato, Yellow	G	G	G
Pumpkin	G	G	G
Radishes	R	O	Y
Shallots	R	R	Y
Spaghetti Squash	G	B	B

Spinach	O	Y	B
Squash, Butternut	G	B	B
Sugar Snap Peas	R	O	Y
Sweet Potato	Y	Y	B
Swiss Chard	R	O	Y
Tomatillo	R	O	Y
Tomato	R	O	Y
Turnip	R	O	Y
Yam Root	Y	O	Y
Zucchini	B	G	G

HERBS

During Flares

1. Remember to eat herbs in blue color in moderation during flares.
2. It is fine to boil or steam herbs and consume during flares.
3. Check if an herb is easy to digest or not. If it is hard to digest, avoid eating it during flares.
4. Check if an herb has anti-inflammatory properties or not. Consider other factors when you chose an herb to consume during flares.

During Remissions

1. Many herbs can be well-tolerated during remission periods.
2. Use more herbs with anti-inflammatory properties and rich in nutrients and vitamins required for IBD patients during remission periods.

Table 4. List of herbs to eat and to avoid

Herbs:	Flare-up	Remission
Aloe Vera	R	G
Angelica	Y	G
Basil	Y	G
Bay	Y	G

Bee Balm	R	B
Calendula	Y	G
Caraway	R	B
Catnip	R	B
Cayenne	R	R
Chamomile	Y	G
Chives	R	B
Cilantro	R	B
Cinnamon	G	G
Coriander	R	B
Dill	R	B
Fennel	R	B
Garlic	R	O
Geraniums	R	B
Ginger	G	G
Ginseng	B	G
Hibiscus	R	B
Horseradish	R	B
Laurel	R	B
Lavender	Y	B
Lemon Balm	Y	B
Lemongrass	O	B
Lemon Zest	Y	G
Licorice Root	O	B
Marjoram	R	B
Milk Thistle	R	B
Mint	Y	G
Nettle	Y	G
Oregano	O	G
Parsley	O	B
Peppermint	Y	G
Rosemary	Y	G
Saffron	Y	G
Sage	R	B
Salvia	R	B
Savory	R	B
Sweet bay	R	B
Sweet cicely	R	B
Sweetgrass	R	B
Tarragon	R	B
Thyme	Y	G
Tulsi / Holy Basil	Y	G
Turmeric	G	G
Yarrow	R	B

SPICES

During Flares

1. Do not forget to consume spices in blue color in moderation during flares.
2. Check if a spice is hot and spicy. If yes, avoid consuming it during flares.
3. Check if a spice has anti-inflammatory properties or not. Consider other factors when you chose a spice to use during flares.

During Remissions

1. Many spices can be well-tolerated during remission periods.
2. Use more herbs with anti-inflammatory properties and rich in nutrients and vitamins required for IBD patients during remission periods.

Table 5. List of spices to eat and to avoid

Spices:	Flare-up	Remission
Angelica	Y	G
Bay leaf	Y	G
Basil	Y	G
Bergamot	Y	G
Black cumin	O	G
Black pepper	R	Y
Burnet	Y	G
Caraway	R	B
Cardamom	Y	G
Catnip	R	B
Cayenne pepper	R	R
Chicory	O	G
Chili pepper	R	R
Chives	R	B
Cicely	O	G
Cilantro	R	B
Cinnamon	G	G

Clove	R	B
Coriander	R	B
Cumin	Y	G
Curry	R	B
Dill	R	B
Fennel	R	B
Fenugreek	R	B
Ginger	G	G
Holy basil	Y	B
Horseradish	R	B
Lavender	Y	B
Lemon balm	Y	B
Lemongrass	O	B
Licorice	O	B
Marjoram	R	B
Nutmeg	R	B
Oregano	Y	G
Paprika	R	O
Parsley	Y	B
Peppermint	Y	G
Poppyseed	R	B
Rosemary	Y	G
Saffron	Y	G
Sage	R	B
Salt	G	G
Sesame	R	O
Spearmint	Y	G
Sumac	Y	B
Tarragon	R	B
Thyme	Y	G
Turmeric	G	G
Vanilla	Y	G

OILS

During Flares

1. It is highly recommended to avoid consuming lots of oil during flare-up periods. Most meals should be boiled or cooked without consuming oils.
2. A safe option for cooking during flares is using extra virgin olive oil in moderation.

3. Avocado and fish oils are also other safe options.

During Remissions

1. Patients can consume most cooking oils during remission periods. However, it is recommended to avoid consuming palm and corn oils.
2. Always try to consume high-quality organic oils.
3. Remember that the best options are extra virgin olive oil and avocado oil.
4. Check your tolerance if you want to cook your meal with any of the oils shown in yellow in the table below.

Table 6. List of oils to eat and to avoid

Cooking Oils/Fats	Flare-up	Remission
Butter	R	Y
Olive Oil	B	G
Extra Virgin Olive Oil	G	G
Coconut Oil	R	Y
Animal Fats	R	O
Palm Oil	R	O
Avocado Oil	G	G
Fish Oil	B	G
Flax Oil	R	Y
Canola Oil	O	Y
Nut Oils and Peanut Oil	**Flare-up**	**Remission**
Peanut oil	R	Y
Macadamia nut oil	Y	G
Seed and Vegetable Oils	**Flare-up**	**Remission**
Soybean oil	R	Y
Corn oil	R	O
Cottonseed oil	R	Y
Rapeseed oil	R	Y
Sunflower oil	R	Y
Sesame oil	R	Y
Grapeseed oil	R	B
Safflower oil	R	Y
Rice bran oil	R	Y

ANIMAL PROTEINS

During Flares

1. Avoid eating skins and fat cuts.
2. Avoid eating cold cuts.
3. Avoid eating spicy cold cuts.
4. Avoid eating hard to digest meats.
5. Avoid eating animal proteins with the skin.
6. Eat animal proteins shown in blue color in moderation.
7. Use lean or extra lean cuts for red meat and pork if you can tolerate them during flares.
8. The ostrich is an excellent source of protein to try during flares.
9. Poaching and boiling eggs are the best methods of making eggs during flare-up periods. Do not consume fried eggs during flares.

During Remissions

1. Remove skins of poultries and other animal proteins before consumption.
2. Stick to lean and extra lean cuts during remission periods as well.
3. Remember to eat animal proteins in blue in moderation.
4. Try to limit red meats in your meal plan.
5. Put high amounts of animal proteins in your weekly meal plan.
6. Avoid consuming fatty parts of meat, chicken, and pork during remission periods, as well.

Table 7. List of animal proteins to eat and to avoid

Animal Proteins	Flare-up	Remission
Red Meat:		
Beef	R	Y
Bison	R	Y

Goat leans	R	Y
Lamb	R	Y
Moose	R	Y
Ostrich	B	G
Venison	R	Y
Veal	R	Y
Kangaroo	R	Y
Lean/Extra Lean Red Meat	B	G
Eggs:		
Chicken eggs	B	G
Quail eggs	B	G
Poultry:		
Chicken	G	G
Turkey	G	G
Duck	G	G
Goose	G	G
Pork:		
Pork	R	O
Ham	R	O
Bacon	R	O
Pork Lean	B	G
Pork Tenderloin	B	G
Other:		
Sausage	R	O
Pepperoni	R	O
Salami	R	O

SEAFOOD

1. Seafood is an excellent source of healthy fatty acids for patients.
2. Always (during flares or remissions) put seafood in your weekly meal plan.
3. Remember to consume seafood shown in blue color in moderation during flare-up periods.
4. It is recommended to avoid consuming scallops or caviars during flare-up periods.

Table 8. List of seafood to eat and to avoid

Seafood	Flare-up	Remission
Tuna	G	G

Salmon	G	G
Trout	G	G
Bluefish	G	G
Catfish	G	G
Halibut	G	G
Clams	B	G
Oyster	B	G
Mussels	B	G
Crab	G	G
Lobster	G	G
Shrimps	G	G
Prawns	G	G
Scallop	O	B
Caviar	O	B

WHOLE GRAINS

1. It is recommended not to consume whole grains during flare-up periods at all. Oatmeal can be checked and then, consumed during flares.
2. During remission, consuming whole grains depend on the health condition of a patient. If a patient has a complication such as strictures, or a part of large intestine surgically removed, she/he needs to avoid whole grains.
3. It is also recommended for other patients to avoid consuming whole grains in the remission period as well. Oatmeal family and quinoa are excluded from this rule. They can be consumed in moderation if they can be tolerated well.

Table 9. List of whole grains to eat and to avoid

Whole Grains	Flare-up	Remission
Amaranth	R	O
Barley	O	Y
Brown Rice	R	O
Brown Rice Bread	R	O
Brown Rice Tortilla	R	O
Buckwheat	R	O
Bulgur (Cracked Wheat)	R	O

Farro / Emmer	R	O
Flaxseed	R	O
Grano	R	O
Kamut / Khorasan	R	Y
Millet	R	O
Oats	O	Y
Oat Bread	O	Y
Oat Cereal	O	Y
Oatmeal	Y	B
Popcorn	R	R
Whole Wheat Cereal Flakes	R	O
Muesli	R	O
Rolled Oats	R	B
Quinoa	R	Y
Rye	R	O
Sorghum	R	O
Spelt	R	O
Teff	R	O
Triticale	R	O
Whole Grain Barley	R	O
Wheat Berries	R	O
Whole Grain Cornmeal	R	O
Whole Rye	R	O
Whole Wheat Bread	R	O
Whole Wheat Couscous	R	O
Whole Wheat Crackers	R	O
Whole Wheat Pasta	R	O
Whole Wheat Pita Bread	R	O
Whole Wheat Sandwich Buns And Rolls	R	O
Whole Wheat Tortillas	R	O
Wild Rice	R	O

REFINED GRAINS

1. Some of the white refined grains such as white rice, macaroni, and pasta can be well-tolerated during flare-up periods. Hence, consider them in your flare-up meal plan.
2. Most of the white grains can be well-tolerated during remission periods.

3. It is recommended not to consume grain products with corn.
4. It is recommended to consume organic, non-GMO grains.

Table 10. List of refined grains to eat and to avoid

Refined Grains	Flare-up	Remission
Cornbread	R	O
Corn Tortillas	R	O
Couscous	O	Y
Crackers	O	G
Flour Tortillas	O	B
Noodles	B	G
Spaghetti	B	G
Macaroni	B	G
Pitas	B	G
Pretzels	Y	Y
Ready-To-Eat Breakfast Cereals	O	Y
White Bread	B	G
White Sandwich Buns and Rolls	B	G
White Rice	G	G

GLUTEN-FREE FLOUR OPTIONS

1. Many gluten-free flours may not be tolerated well during remission periods. It is recommended to avoid consuming them if it is possible.
2. On the contrary, many gluten-free flour options can be well-tolerated during remission periods, but it is recommended to consume gluten-free flours without whole grains.
3. Flours from nuts should be well-grounded.
4. Do not consume flours with high non-soluble fibers during flares.

Table 11. Gluten-free flours to eat and to avoid

Gluten-Free Flours	Flare-up	Remission

Almond Flour	Y	G
Buckwheat Flour	O	Y
Sorghum Flour	O	Y
Amaranth Flour	O	Y
Teff Flour	O	Y
Arrowroot Flour	Y	B
Brown Rice Flour	R	O
Oat Flour	Y	B
Corn Flour	R	O
Chickpea Flour	R	Y
Coconut Flour	R	Y
Tapioca Flour	O	B
Cassava Flour	O	B
Tigernut Flour	R	B

NUTS

During Flares

1. It is highly recommended to avoid consuming raw nuts during flare-up periods.

During Remissions

1. Remission2: Some patients without having intestine complications can consume limited amounts of nuts. It is recommended for this group to check their tolerance regarding each type of nuts they want to eat.
2. Remission1: It is highly recommended for patients with large intestine complications such as strictures, or any other complications from the large intestine surgeries, to avoid consuming nuts during flares and remission periods.
3. Some nuts such as almond can be used in moderation in other formats such as smoothened almond butter or almond milk and if they can be well-tolerated.

4. Make sure the almond butter or other nut butter you want to consume is smooth.
5. You can also make stews with well-ground nuts if you can tolerate them.

Table 12. List of nuts to eat and to avoid: Remission1 patients with colon complications, Remission2: typical IBD patients

Nuts	Flare-up	Remission1	Remission2
Almond	R	O	B
Black Walnut	R	O	Y
Brazil Nut	R	O	Y
Butternut	R	O	Y
Candlenut	R	O	Y
Cashew	R	O	B
Chestnuts	R	O	Y
Hazelnut	R	O	Y
Hickory Nut	R	O	Y
Macadamia	R	O	Y
Oak Acorns	R	O	Y
Pecan	R	O	Y
Persian Walnuts	R	O	Y
Pine Nut	R	O	Y
Pistachio	R	O	Y
Walnut	R	O	Y
White Nut	R	O	Y

SEEDS

During Flares

1. It is highly recommended to avoid consuming seeds during flare-up periods.

During Remissions

1. Remission2: Some patients without having intestine complications can consume limited amounts of seeds. It is recommended for this group to check their tolerance regarding each type of seeds they want to eat.

2. Remission1: It is highly recommended for patients with large intestine complications such as strictures, or any other complications from the large intestine surgeries, to avoid consuming seeds during flares and remission periods.

Table 13. List of seeds to eat and to avoid: Remission1 patients with colon complications, Remission2: typical IBD patients

Seeds	Flare-up	Remission1	Remission2
Chia seeds	R	O	Y
Flaxseed	R	O	Y
Hemp seeds	R	O	Y
Poppyseed	R	O	Y
Pumpkin seeds	R	O	Y
Sesame seed	R	O	Y
Safflower	R	O	Y
Sunflower	R	O	Y

LEGUMES

1. Avoid consuming legumes during flares.
1. It is recommended not to consume legumes highlighted in orange color even during remission.
2. Check your tolerance level when you want to consume legumes shown in yellow color.
3. You may consume green peas in moderation during remission periods.

Table 14. List of legumes to eat and to avoid

Legumes	Flare-up	Remission
Adzuki beans	R	O
Black beans	R	O
Soybeans	R	Y
Anasazi beans	R	O
Fava beans	R	Y
Chickpeas	R	Y
Kidney beans	R	O
Lima beans	R	O
Peanut	R	O
Green peas	R	B

Snow peas	R	Y
Snap peas	R	Y
Split peas	R	O
Black-eyed peas	R	O
Yellow lentils	R	O
Orange lentils	R	O
Green lentils	R	O
Brown lentils	R	O
Black lentils	R	O

SWEETENERS

During Flares

1. It is highly recommended to avoid consuming artificial sweeteners during flare-up periods.
2. White sugar needs to be significantly limited during flare-up periods.
3. Patients need to check their tolerance for sweeteners such as honey or maple syrup.
4. It seems that Stevia can be well-tolerated. However, use it in moderation during flare-up periods.

During Remissions

1. It is recommended to avoid consuming artificial sweeteners, even during remission periods.
2. It is recommended to consume natural sugars or plant-based sweeteners during remission periods such as stevia (instead of white processed sugar).
3. Honey, maple syrup, molasses, and stevia seem to be some promising options for white processed sugar. Make sure you can tolerate them well.

Table 15. List of sweeteners

Sweeteners	Flare-up	Remission	Notes:
Acesulfame K	R	O	Artificial Sweetener

Agave Syrup	Y	Y	Modified Sugar
Aspartame	R	O	Artificial Sweetener
Brown Sugar	R	Y	Sugar
Cane Juice	R	Y	Sugar Extract
Caramel	R	O	Modified Sugar
Coconut Sugar	R	B	Sugar Extract
Corn Sugar (HFCS)	R	R	Modified Sugar
Corn Sweetener (HFCS)	R	R	Modified Sugar
Corn Syrup (HFCS)	R	R	Modified Sugar
Curcumin	R	B	Natural Sweetener
Dextrose	R	O	Sugar
Erythritol	R	Y	Sugar Alcohol
Fructose Glucose Syrup (HFCS)	R	R	Modified Sugar
Glucitol (Sorbitol)	R	R	Sugar Alcohol
Glucose-Fructose Syrup (HFCS)	R	R	Modified Sugar
Golden Syrup	R	R	Modified Sugar
High Fructose Corn Syrup (HFCS)	R	R	Modified Sugar
Honey	Y	B	Natural Sugar
Mannitol	R	Y	Sugar Alcohol
Maple Syrup	Y	B	Sugar Extract
Molasses	O	B	Sugar Extract
Palm Sugar	R	O	Sugar Extract
Saccharin	R	O	Artificial Sweetener
Sorbitol	R	Y	Sugar Alcohol
Stevia, Aka Truvia or Pure Via	B	G	Natural Sweetener
Sucralose	R	O	Artificial Sweetener
White sugar (Table Sugar)	O	B	Sugar: Sucrose
Xylitol	R	Y	Sugar Alcohol

DAIRY PRODUCTS

During Flares

1. It is highly recommended to avoid consuming dairy products during flare-up periods as these products are hard to digest and can irritate your gut.

During Remissions

1. Some patients without lactose intolerance are typically able to consume milk, goat milk, kefir, yogurt, yogurt drinks, or other types of dairies during remission periods in moderation. This group of patients needs to avoid consuming fatty cheese even during remission. It is also recommended for this group of patients to put yogurt and kefir in their meal plan as they are excellent sources of probiotics and prebiotics, respectively.
2. Lactose-intolerant patients need to avoid consuming dairy products with lactose, even during remission periods.

Table 16. List of dairy products to eat and to avoid

Dairy	Flare-up	Lactose Intolerant Flare	Remission	Lactose Intolerant Remission
Milk	R	R	Y	R
Goat milk	R	O	B	O
Fermented Milk	R	R	Y	R
Kefir	O	R	G	R
Yogurt	R	R	G	R
Yogurt drinks	R	R	G	R
Cream	R	R	Y	R
Sour cream	R	R	Y	R
Fatty Cheese	R	R	O	R

LACTOSE-FREE YOGURT PRODUCTS

During Flares

1. It is highly recommended to avoid consuming yogurt products during flare-up periods.

During Remissions

1. Lactose-intolerant patients can consume lactose-free yogurt options according to Table 18 below:

Table 17. List of lactose-free yogurt products to eat and to avoid

Lactose-Free Yogurt	Flare-up	Remission
Soy Yogurt	R	Y
Lactose-free yogurt	R	G
Almond milk yogurt	O	G
Coconut milk yogurt	R	Y
Cashewgurt	R	Y
Nut yogurt (plant-based yogurt)	R	Y

BUTTER

During Flares

1. It is highly recommended to avoid consuming butter during flare-up periods.

During Remissions

1. Patients in remission can consume butter in moderation. However, it is recommended to check your tolerance when consuming it.
2. It is also recommended not to consume salted butter.
3. The best-recommended butter option for those who can tolerate butter during remission periods is organic grass-fed butter.

Table 18. List of butter to eat and to avoid

Butter	Flare-up	Remission
Salted Butter	R	O
Unsalted Butter	R	Y

Grass-fed Butter	R	B
Margarine	R	O

LACTOSE-FREE MILK PRODUCTS

During Flares

1. It is highly recommended to avoid consuming milk products during flare-up periods.

During Remissions

1. Lactose-intolerant patients can consume lactose-free milk options according to the below table. They need to check alternative options to the cow milk to see if they do not have any problem consuming them.

Table 19. List of lactose-free milk products to eat and to avoid

Lactose-Free Milk	Flare-up	Remission
Almond Milk	O	G
Soy Milk	R	Y
Cashew Milk	R	Y
Rice Milk	O	G
Coconut Milk	R	Y
Hemp Milk	R	Y
Pea Milk	R	Y
Oat Milk	R	G
Peanut Milk	R	O
Flax Milk	R	Y
Walnut Milk	R	Y

CHEESES

During Flares

1. It is highly recommended to avoid consuming cheese products during flare-up periods as cheeses are hard to digest foods and can irritate the gut.

During Remissions

1. Patients who are not lactose-intolerant can consume cheese options according to the below table. They need to check cheese types and see if they can tolerate them or not.
2. For patients who are lactose intolerant, there are varieties of lactose-free options shown in blue to consume. For cheeses shown in yellow color, patients need to check if they can tolerate them or not.
3. It is recommended for patients who are not lactose intolerant to consume lactose-free cheese options as well.
4. It is recommended not to consume soft and fatty cheeses, even during remission periods.

Table 20. List of cheeses to eat and to avoid

Hard Cheeses	Flare-up	Remission
Asiago	R	Y
Blue	R	Y
Bra	R	Y
Buffalo	R	Y
Four Herb Gouda	R	Y
Halloumi	R	Y
Jarlsberg	R	Y
Marble Cheddar	O	Y
Monterey Jack Dry	R	O
Parmesan (Parmigiano)	O	B
Parmigiano Reggiano	O	B
Pecorino	O	B
Pecorino Romano	O	B
Reggianito	O	Y
Romano	R	Y
Seriously Strong Cheddar	O	Y
Smoked Gouda	R	Y
Swiss	O	B
Yaroslavsky	R	Y
Semi-Hard Cheese		
Canadian Cheddar	R	O
Cheddar	R	O

Gouda	R	O
Monterey Jack	R	O
Provolone	R	O
Sweet Style Swiss	O	Y
Yorkshire Blue	R	O
Semi-Soft Cheese	R	O
American Cheese	R	O
Baby Swiss	R	Y
Bocconcini	R	O
Cream Havarti	R	O
Low Fat Feta	R	Y
Fresh Jack	R	O
Fromage de Montagne de Savoie	R	O
Havarti	O	Y
Monastery Cheeses	R	O
Mozzarella (Australian)	R	O
Paneer	R	O
Pasteurized Processed	R	O
Soft Cheese		
Ambert	R	O
Brie	R	O
Broccio	R	O
Broccio Demi-Affine	R	O
Cottage Cheese	R	O
Cream Cheese	R	O
Feta	R	O
Fresh Mozzarella	R	O
Fresh Ricotta	R	O
Fruit Cream Cheese	R	O
Gorgonzola	R	O
Labneh	R	O
Mascarpone	R	O
Mozzarella	R	O
Mozzarella in water	R	O
Ricotta	R	O
Goat Cheese	R	Y

SAUCES, DIPS, AND GRAVIES

During Flares

1. Avoid eating greasy and fatty sauces/gravies.

2. Avoid eating spicy sauces/gravies.
3. Avoid consuming high sugar gravies/sauces.
4. Avoid eating sauces or gravies with triggering ingredients such as onions.
5. Avoid eating hard to digest sauces/gravies.
6. Avoid eating gravies/sauces with nuts and seeds inside.
7. Remember to eat ready gravies/sauces in blue in moderation.
8. Avoid consuming sauces/gravies with milk inside during flares.

During Remissions

1. Eat gravies/sauces in green and blue in moderation.
2. Always make healthy and fresh gravies/sauces.
3. It is recommended to consume low-fat, low-sodium organic sauces.
4. Avoid spicy sauces/gravies even during remission periods.

Table 21. List of sauces to eat and to avoid

Sauces, and Dips	Flare-up	Remission
BBQ	R	B
Apple Cider Vinegar	R	O
French dip	R	B
Ketchup	R	O
Mayonnaise	O	Y
Honey Garlic	R	Y
Tomato sauce	R	O
Hot sauce	R	R
Peppercorn sauce	R	R
Sour cream sauce	R	B
Mustard	R	O
Sweet chili		
Tartar sauce	Y	B
Vinaigrette	Y	G
Wine sauce	R	O
Worcestershire sauce	R	B

Gravy	Y	B
Mushroom gravy	R	
Poutine	R	B
Thousand island	R	B
Tobasco	R	R
Onion sauce	R	O
Salsa	R	O
Applesauce	G	G
Cranberry sauce	R	Y
Mango sauce	Y	B
Strawberry sauce	R	Y
Balsamic	Y	B
White vinegar	R	B
Red vinegar	R	B
Sour grape	R	B
Béchamel sauce	Y	B
Oyster sauce	R	B
Soy sauce	Y	B
Teryaki sauce	R	B
Tzatziki	R	Y
Pesto	R	Y
Alfredo	R	B
Arrabbiata sauce	R	O
Marinara sauce	R	O
Café de Paris sauce	R	Y
Sweet chili sauce	R	R
Garlic sauce	R	O
Guacamole sauce	R	B
Mushroom sauce	R	Y
Cheez whiz	R	Y
Cheddar sauce	R	Y
Butter chicken	R	Y

READY FOODS (IN GENERAL)

During Flares

1. Avoid eating greasy and fatty foods (e.g., fast foods).
2. Avoid eating spicy foods.
3. Avoid eating foods with triggering ingredients.
4. Avoid eating hard to digest foods.
5. Avoid eating foods with lots of sugar.

6. Avoid eating processed and canned foods.
7. Avoid eating foods with high insoluble fiber.
8. Avoid eating foods with nuts and seeds inside.
9. Remember to eat ready foods shown in blue color in moderation.
10. It's better to eat low residue, low fiber foods during flares.

During Remissions

1. Always try to consume fresh and healthy foods.
2. Foods with healthy fats are also suitable for IBD patients.
3. Foods rich in soluble fiber and high in protein are excellent choices during remission periods.
4. Avoid eating spicy foods and triggering foods, even during remission periods.
5. You can have meals with sugar, but make sure that the sugar has been used moderately in the meals you want to eat.

Table 22. List of ready foods

Ready Foods	Flare-up	Remission
Applesauce	G	G
Bruschetta	R	Y
Bagels	R	B
Bisque	Y	G
Babaganoosh	R	Y
Burrito	R	O
Butter chicken	R	Y
Cake	R	B
Candy	R	B
Carne Asada	R	B
Cheeseburger	R	O
Chimichanga	R	O
Chips	R	Y
Chocolate	R	O
Chocolate Bars	R	O
Chowder	O	B

Cookies	R	B
Cupcakes	R	B
Curry	R	Y
Dumplings	Y	B
Donuts	R	Y
Enchilada	R	O
Eggrolls	Y	B
English muffins	R	B
Eel sushi	O	B
Fajita	R	B
Falafel	R	Y
Frankfurters	R	R
Fried Chicken	R	Y
Fondu	R	O
French onion soup	R	O
Gnocchi	B	G
Granola	R	B
Guacamole	R	B
Gumbo	R	Y
Grits	R	O
Graham crackers	O	B
Hamburgers	R	O
Hash browns	R	B
HFCS Products	R	O
Huenos Rancheros	R	Y
Hotdogs	R	O
Hummus	Y	G
Ice cream	R	B
Irish stew	R	Y
Indian food	R	O
Italian bread	R	Y
Kabobs	G	G
Jambalaya	R	O
Jelly/jam	R	Y
Jerky	R	Y
Lasagna	R	Y
Marshmallow	O	B
Meatballs	R	Y
Noodles	Y	Y
Charcuterie	R	O
Pizza	R	Y
Pancakes	R	Y
Quesadilla	R	Y
Quiche	R	Y
Reuben	R	Y

Rice Noodles	B	G
Sashimi	Y	G
Sorbet	Y	G
Sushi	Y	B
Tater tots	R	O
Waffles	R	B
White steamed rice	G	G
Ziti	R	Y
Zucchini Chips	B	G

Chapter 3. How to Cook in Low Residue Diet

Each patient with a gastrointestinal disorder is unique in terms of symptoms, complications, food intolerances, and sensitivities. That is why there is not a single diet for everyone. However, there are essential points that need to be taken into account when you want to cook for a patient:

Cooking Styles/Methods

1. The best cooking methods for patients who wants to follow the low residue diet are boiling, steaming, roasting, grilling, poaching, stewing, and air frying.
2. It is crucial not to fry (especially deep fry) foods during flare-up periods. If you want to fry, simmer or cook on a pan, use a small amount of extra virgin olive oil. Even you can spray it when roasting or grilling.
3. When grilling beef or poultry, make sure the inside of your meat cooked well. Always try to grill well-done.
4. You can poach fruits and boil vegetables and other meals to consume. These are the best cooking methods during flare-ups. If you are poaching fruits, make sure you use small amounts of sugar. We recommend not to use refined sugars at all. If you need a substitute for sugar, you can try stevia. Other possible options are honey, maple syrup, and agave syrup.

Remember to consume these alternatives only if you can tolerate them well.

5. Air frying is the best option if you want to have skin-removed potato chips and zucchini chips. Consume a small amount of extra virgin olive oil when you want to air fry by an air fryer.
6. Broiling is another method that can be fine with many patients. However, patients should avoid eating the burned parts of broiled food.
7. In brief, the best cooking methods for a patient with gastrointestinal disorder such as IBD during a flare are boiling/poaching and steaming. During remission, other cooking styles can be used by consuming a moderate amount of oil. The recommended oil to use is an extra virgin olive oil (if available, buy high-quality organic one).

Food Ingredients

Fruits and Vegetables

Fruits and vegetables contain valuable sources of nutrients that are essential. When you have inflammation in your GI tract, you need to make sure that you eat fruits and vegetables that are very easy to digest.

1. Remember that during the remission period, patients can have certain raw fruits such as apple and pear. However, the skin should be removed. Making a fruit salad from these fruits is a great meal option.
2. During a severe flare-up, it is recommended to consume skin-removed poached/boiled fruits

instead of raw fruits with no sugar or a tiny amount of it (if it can be tolerated).
3. During a severe flare-up, boil or steam vegetables that are easier to digest, such as asparagus and skin-removed potatoes.
4. Making a vegetable broth or stock is a great meal option.
5. Avoid fruit and vegetable seeds.
6. Avoid juices with the pulp.
7. The best option for juicing fruits and vegetables is to use a sturdy juicer or a juicing machine. When you are juicing with such devices, you are removing the fibers of fruits and vegetables. As such, you can get vitamins, minerals, and other healthy properties of fruits and vegetables without getting their fiber. This approach is fabulous for patients with large intestine narrowing or strictures or any other patients who should follow a low-fiber diet.
8. The best fruit and vegetable juices for many patients are banana, cantaloupe, melon, papaya, apple, lemon, watermelon, squash (no seeds), pumpkin, cucumber, pomegranate, carrot, celery, zucchini, and cucumber.

Rice, Noodle and Pasta

1. Try not to consume wild rice and brown rice. The best rice option for patients is white rice, such as basmati or Jasmine white rice.
2. To make an excellent rice meal, steamed white rice in a rice maker or a proper pot.

3. The best noodle option for you is Asian-style rice noodles as they are low in fiber and can be cooked so fast.
4. Another great noodle for you is egg noodles. This type of noodle is low in fiber as well, which is excellent for patients that need to follow a low-residue diet.
5. Alternatively, you can make zucchini noodles or spiralized zucchini using a spiralizer.
6. Cook your pasta according to its package instruction. Typically, you need to choose a proper pot and pour water on top of your pasta to cover all pasta. After boiling water, cook pasta in the boiling water for about 10 minutes. You can add salt and extra virgin olive oil to the boiling water to taste. Use them in moderation.
7. If you are not a gluten-intolerant patient, you can cook most of the regular pasta with gluten, but remember to use whole wheat or whole grain pasta in moderation.
8. If you are a gluten-intolerant patient, you can have gluten-free pasta with white rice flour or soy. You can have other types of gluten-free pasta such as quinoa or brown rice in moderation and check if you can tolerate them.
9. Alternatively, you can make spaghetti squash to have a delicious vegetarian spaghetti.

Meat and Poultry

Animal proteins contain various types of vitamins and minerals, such as vitamin-B, E, zinc, magnesium, and iron. They also have amino acids that are essential for IBD patients. That is why IBD patients need to eat varieties of animal proteins. Moreover, they need to take more protein during flare-up periods to increase the time of recovery from inflammation.

1. Do not use processed meats at all. Consuming meats that have been salted, fermented, smoked, or canned is not recommended. Avoid consuming cold-cuts and sausage products.
2. Reduce the amount of red meat you eat every week.
3. When in remission, you can have extra lean or lean red meat in moderation. Choose low-fat or no-fat cuts.
4. During a flare-up, you need to limit your red meat intake. Just use no-fat well-cooked extra lean (or lean) part or avoid consuming red meat if you are experiencing a severe flare.
5. Do not stir fry meat and poultry when you are in a flare. Cook them well in boiling water.
6. Avoid consuming fatty parts of any meat.
7. Ostrich meat without fat is one of the best red meat options for patients. The ostrich meat has a similar taste of beef meat, but with lower fat and cholesterol. Moreover, it is rich in protein, iron, and calcium that are fantastic for IBD patients.
8. Do not eat spicy or fatty meat products such as salami and pepperoni during flare-up periods.
9. You can cook chicken/turkey breasts, legs, and thighs. Make sure the skins are removed. It is not recommended to eat chicken wings during a flare.
10. Limit the usage of pork. Use low-fat (or no fat) extra lean (or lean) part of pork meat.
11. Avoid eating bacon during flares. Limit eating it during remission, as well.

SEAFOOD

Seafood is another excellent source of protein, amino acids, and healthy fats. Oily fish contain healthful fats, including omega-3 fatty acids. This combat inflammation and may help reduce the risk of heart disease and certain cancers. Health experts often recommend eating at least two servings of oily fish per week. These can include trout, salmon, mackerel, herring, tuna, and sardines.

1. To keep fat levels as low as possible, grill the fish or bake them with small amounts of extra virgin olive oil. It is the best way to cook the fish, for easy digestion.
2. Tuna is another excellent seafood that patient may want to consume. You can make a delicious sandwich with tuna, avocado, and lemon juice. It is not recommended to eat raw sashimi such as tuna sashimi, especially if you are not sure about the place you purchased them, as you will be more vulnerable to diseases such as salmonella.
3. Well-cooked shrimps, prawns, and crabs can also be consumed in remission and flare periods.

GRAINS

Grains are excellent sources of fiber, vitamin-B, iron, and other healthy nutrients such as magnesium and selenium. In general, grains contain three components: germ, bran, and endosperm. Whole grains have all three components, but refined grains have a process of removing the germ and bran to have a smooth texture. During this process, some iron and B-vitamin can be removed from the grain. As such, some recommend consuming whole grain products during remission if you can tolerate and if you are entirely sure that you do not have any complications such as stricture in your large intestine. Otherwise, use refined grains.

1. Refined grains have less fermentable fiber than whole grains, so they pass more quickly through the digestive tract. They tend to be easier on the gut and less likely to cause inflammation.
2. Examples of refined grains include: white bread, white rice, pasta, plain crackers, pancakes, waffles, and rice snacks.
3. All-purpose white flour is an excellent option for cooking and baking. Alternatively, almond flour is another superb option for IBD patients, especially for those who are gluten intolerant.
4. Ready-to-eat cereals that are low in fiber are also a good option. Also, fortified refined grains contain added essential nutrients, such as as vitamins and minerals. So, a person should look for fortified products. Many breads, for example, are fortified with iodine and folate. Manufacturers also tend to fortify ready-to-eat cereals with vitamins A, C, and D, thiamine, iron, and folate.
5. Remember that gluten-intolerant patients need to avoid gluten and alternatively consume non-triggering gluten-free products.
6. The oatmeal made from quick or rolled oats is a type of refined grain, with slightly less fiber than steel-cut oats. Manufacturers produce oats by removing the hulls. When experiencing a flare-up, it is best to avoid foods containing insoluble fiber, which can worsen symptoms of diarrhea. Oatmeal contains a soluble fiber called beta-glucan. It can help ease diarrhea by absorbing water in the intestines, forming a gel, slowing digestion, and adding bulk to stool.

7. Try adding oats to smoothies that contain peeled, low-fiber fruits. Breaking down food in a blender makes digestion easier. However, if you see that you cannot tolerate oatmeal well during a severe flare-up, avoid consuming it.

SOY, EGGS, AND FIRM TOFU

1. Soy, eggs, and tofu are great sources of lean protein. Also, egg yolks contain high amounts of vitamin D, and people with IBD are often deficient in vitamin D and A.
2. In addition to lean protein, soy and tofu contain bioactive peptides, and some research suggests that these have antioxidant and anti-inflammatory properties, which may help manage your disease.
3. Do not eat fried eggs or scrambled eggs during a flare-up. Alternatively, hard-boil eggs.
4. When you are in a flare, bake tofu instead of stir-frying it.

DAIRY PRODUCTS

1. Many yogurts contain probiotics, which are healthful bacteria that may help reduce inflammation in the gut.
2. Dairy products are rich in calcium, and manufacturers may fortify them with vitamins D and C. Many, however, contain lactose, a type of sugar, and some doctors recommend eliminating lactose from the diet. The number of dairy servings per day may depend upon the individual dietary needs of a person with Crohn's. As explained, some people with the condition find dairy products worsen their

symptoms. If not the case, a person can eat two servings or less of the following options:
- Cheese
- Cottage cheese
- Milk
- Yogurt with live active cultures

3. Lactose-intolerant patients should avoid any forms of lactose in their cooking. It is also recommended for patients that are not lactose intolerant to limit consuming dairy products while in flare-up as generally, dairy products are hard to be digested. Suggested alternatives are:
- Almond milk
- Oat milk
- Soy milk
- Rice milk

SPICES AND HERBS

1- Certain spices can be used in your cooking. Turmeric, ginger, and cinnamon are great spices for meals as they have anti-inflammation and anti-microbial properties.
2- Salt can also be consumed. As a general health recommendation, use it in moderation.
3- Black pepper can only be used during remission periods in moderation.
4- Other hot spicy peppers such as cayenne or red pepper are not recommended.
5- Do not use garlic powder as well.
6- Try not to use onion powder as well.
7- It is recommended to grate ginger instead of mincing it.

8- Other recommended herbs that can be used in moderation are: thyme, oregano, and saffron
9- Lemon zest can be used during remission in moderation.
10- Some studies show anti-inflammatory properties of ginseng, as well. You may want to use it in moderation if you can tolerate it well.
11- Use other common herbs such as basil, cilantro, rosemary, Angelica, and parsley in moderation if you can tolerate. Try not to consume during a severe flare-up or use a small number of cooked versions.

Cheese

1- If you can tolerate lactose, you can consume low-fat cheeses such as feta and cheddar during remission in moderation.
2- It is recommended to limit your cheese intake when you are experiencing a flare-up. It does not matter if you are lactose intolerant or not.
3- If you are lactose-intolerant, you still can have a variety of cheese to consume. Many of patients with lactose intolerance can tolerate cheese with less than 0.5-gram lactose per serving in their meals. Some of the safe cheese to consume for lactose intolerant patients are:
    - Lactose-free Swiss
    - Hard grating cheeses such as Parmigiano-Reggiano and Pecorino
    - Aged cheddar
    - Muenster
    - Aged Brie or Camembert

The abovementioned cheeses typically have less than 2% lactose in their servings, which can be tolerated by most lactose-intolerant patients. Some other cheeses with more percentage of lactose are listed below. These cheeses can also be safe (if taken in moderation) for some lactose-intolerant patients. Always check your intolerance level before consuming these cheeses:

- Havarti
- Normal Parmesan
- Provolone
- Gouda
- Blue
- Mild cheddar
- Normal Swiss

Some cheeses to avoid are soft, mozzarellas, fetas, ricottas, and cottages.

Some lactose-intolerant patients can tolerate goat cheeses better. You can check if you can tolerate goat cheese or not.

OILS

1- The best oil recommended is extra virgin olive oil.
2- Avoid consuming butter during flare-ups. Use butter in a minimal amount during remission. The best butter to choose is grass-fed butter.
3- Avocado oil is another recommended oil to use for cooking.
4- Coconut oil is not recommended.
5- Safflower oil, grapeseed oil, sunflower oil, vegetable oil, and soybean oil are other oils that can be used in moderation. They are excellent sources of Omega-6, which is great for the correct inflammatory response.

SAUCE, GRAVY, SALAD DRESSINGS

Here are some of the essential tips for using sauce, gravy, and salad dressings:

- Do not use hot spicy sauces, gravies, or salad dressings.
- Mayonnaise can be used in moderation in remissions only. Try to make or purchase low-fat low-sodium organic types.
- Many of patients cannot tolerate tomato-based products such as Ketchup, tomato sauce, and tomato paste. Check your tolerance level for these types of sauces before consuming them. It is recommended to avoid using them.
- Mustard: avoid using it in general.
- Sour cream: can be used in moderation, but check your tolerance before consuming it.
- Smooth sauces and salad dressings are fine in general. Always try to check your tolerance first, and if you are okay, use them in moderation.
- Gravies: low-sodium low-fat gravies from beef and poultry are generally fine to consume in moderation.
- Soy sauce is fine in general. Always try to check your tolerance first, and if you are okay, use it in moderation.
- Balsamic vinegar: try to check your tolerance first, and if you are okay, only use it in moderation.
- White vinegar: try to check your tolerance first, and if you are okay, only use it in moderation.
- Red/White wines: avoid using wine in sauces or dressings.
- Tahini: is fine in general. Always try to check your tolerance first, and if you are okay, use it in moderation.

- Barbecue (BBQ) sauce: has a high acidity level in it. Check your tolerance first, and if you are okay, use it in moderation.
- Sauces/gravies with garlic or onion: are not recommended.
- Honey and maple syrup are fine in general. Always try to check your tolerance first, and if you are okay, use them in moderation.

DRINKS

Drink options are fully explained in Chapter-10 of this book. In general, patients should avoid sodas, sparkling water, and fizzy beverages. Caffeine should be avoided during a flare-up and limit having caffeinated drinks during remission periods. Some herbal teas such as peppermint and green tea are great alternatives for caffeinated beverages.

MEALS

Breakfast

Breakfast is an essential meal for everyone. Typically, the breakfast of patients who needs to follow the low residue diet should be rich in proteins and soluble fibers. Soluble fibers are easier to digest as they can absorb water and become like gels during the digestion process. Some prefer to consume foods with more carbohydrates in the morning, and some who are more concern about their weight gain want to consume foods with fewer carbohydrates for their breakfast. If you're going to have more carbs, you can consume sweet fruits that are good for patients more. Some of the great breakfast options are:

- Decaffeinated hot drinks (coffee, tea, etc.)
- Eggs: Boiled eggs are recommended.
- Oatmeal: you can combine oatmeal with cinnamon, honey (If you can tolerate), applesauce, or skin-removed cubed apples to have a very delicious oatmeal breakfast.
- Banana oatmeal
- Almond butter (smoothened) sandwich
- Avocado sandwich
- Yogurt and cow milk if you can tolerate and not in a flare.
- Preferably use lactose-free yogurt with skin-removed raw or poached fruits such as papaya, pear, apple, banana during remission.

Soups

Soup is one of the great meals you can have. Perfectly blended soups are very easy to digest and are great for patients who should have a liquid diet or Bland diet, and for patients with complications such as large intestine strictures. Soups can be more in your meal plan during flare-up periods if you can tolerate. Some of the most exceptional soups for patients who wants to follow the low residue diet are:

- Blended bone broth, beef broth, chicken broth, and vegetable broth
- Blended or mashed potato soup (skin-removed)
- Pumpkin soup
- Butternut squash soup
- Chicken noodle soup
- Chicken and white rice soup
- Oatmeal soup

Salads

Salad is a great meal for most people. You can mix different types of foods with different high nutrients, vitamins, and minerals together in a salad. However, making a salad could be a challenging task, as many typical salad ingredients cannot be well-tolerated by the patients. There are lots of different salads for IBD patients. This book provides you with delicious salad recipes in Chapter-10. Some of the fantastic salad options and salad ingredients for IBD patients include but not limited to:

- Skin-removed cucumber and carrot are great salad ingredients for IBD patients.
- Fruit salad can be made from certain fruits IBD patients can tolerate well.
- Many of IBD patients think that they cannot eat salads with lettuce anymore. However, many of IBD patients can tolerate Butter lettuce (or called Bibb lettuce) as this type of lettuce has softer leaves that can be digested easier than other types of lettuces. Try butter lettuce in moderation and check if you can tolerate it or not.
- Zucchini, potato, pasta, and chicken are other great ingredients for having a delicious salad.
- Other salad ingredients such as beets or herbs such as spinach, parsley, and basil might be used in moderation if you can tolerate them. Some IBD patients cannot tolerate vegetables that contain histamine, such as spinach. Always check your tolerance and adjust your diet and meals based on that.

Snacks

Snacks can play a crucial role in the meal plan of IBD patients. IBD patients need to eat smaller portions five or six times during a day. Hence, a full, healthy snack that cannot trigger the disease can be beneficial for IBD patients. Here are some of the snack options for IBD patients:

- Hummus
- Applesauce
- Avocado sandwich
- Gluten-free snacks
- Fruits (poached or compote)
- Rice crackers
- Oatmeal
- Zucchini chips
- Lactose-free milk, such as almond milk
- Cheese sticks (low-fat, lactose-free options)

Avoid consuming chocolates as snacks, especially if you are experiencing a flare-up.

Desserts

Dessert can also be an excellent meal portion for IBD patients to soothe their gut. Here are some of the dessert options for IBD patients:

- Ice creams made with allowed fruits: lactose intolerant patients need to use lactose-free ice creams or sorbets
- Sorbet from allowing fruits
- Shakes made with allowed fruits: lactose intolerant patients need to use lactose-free milk
- Trifle with banana and lemon
- Gluten-free cakes
- Applesauce
- Fruit compote or bowl made with allowed fruits

Side Dishes

Each meal can have its well-matched side dishes. Some of the side dish options for IBD patients include, but not limited to:

- Roasted or boiled potatoes (skin removed)
- Mashed potatoes (recommendations: use olive oil instead of butter and lactose-free milk instead of cow milk if you are lactose-intolerant)
- Boiled vegetables such as spinach (if you can tolerate)
- Zucchini as chips, raw or roasted (skin removed)
- Cooked, raw or glazed carrots
- Mushroom: Check your tolerance first and then consume in moderation if you are fine. If not, you may use shiitake mushroom alternatively.
- Beets: are generally fine. Check your intolerance first and use it in moderation if you can tolerate it.
- Green beans are generally fine. Check your intolerance first and use it in moderation if you can tolerate it.
- Avocado: mashed or cubed
- Lemon or lime wedges
- Well-cooked asparagus or fennel
- Recommendation: try not to use tomatoes, caramelized onion, roasted garlic, raw broccoli, raw cauliflower, and corn.
- Sauerkraut can be consumed in moderation during remissions. You need to avoid consuming it during flares.
- Pickles: Avoid using pickles.

Chapter 4. Food Preparation & Meal Planning

The following tips can help you to have an effective food preparation and meal planning:

Eating Habits

1- Eat smaller portions, but frequent meals 5 to 6 times a day.
2- Keep yourself hydrated. Drink plenty of water and other allowed juices during a day. Pump-up your electrolyte intake, especially during flares using low-sugar sports drinks or use yours at home.
3- Drink slowly and chew well.
4- Do not use straw as you may ingest air, which can cause producing gas.
5- You can drink recommended herbal teas after your meal for better digestion, especially if you think that you ate a lot of your meal was heavy for you.
6- Give time to your herbal tea to brew well.
7- Eat your meal in peace and comfort in a relaxed place. Do not talk too much when you are eating your meal.
8- Do not work with your phone or laptop while eating your meals.
9- Do not drink water in the middle of eating meals.
10- Do not skip your breakfast at all.
11- Do not starve yourself. Determine right specific times for your meals and stick to those times.
12- Do not eat very late. Eat dinner at least 2 hours before your sleep time, or 3 to 4 hours after your lunch.

13- Always have a meal plan and follow it. The worst thing for you is not knowing what to eat and what to cook.
14- Reduce consuming alcohol, sugar, and caffeinated drink. Avoid consuming them in flare-up periods.
15- Do not leave your foods at normal temperature for more than 2 hours.

GROCERY SHOPPING

1- To prepare your meals in advance, you need to create a list before you go to the supermarket for daily or weekly shopping.
2- The list should include ingredients you need for your daily or weekly cooking plan. Remember that the ingredients should be well-tolerated.
3- Always try to purchase organic, non-GMO ingredients
4- Always try to buy lower-fat options.
5- For eggs, try to purchase organic, free-range types
6- For meat or pork, try to pick low-fat lean cuts
7- For poultry, skin-removed breasts and legs are the best options.
8- For cheese, try to purchase low-fat lactose-free options. Use cheese in moderation.
9- For milk and yogurts, always purchase unsweetened and unflavored types.
10- For milk, try to purchase low-fat lactose-free options such as almond milk or rice milk. Use milk in moderation.
11- For grains, try not to get whole-wheat or whole-grain options. Stick to gluten-free options. White breads may also work for you.

12- For bread, try to find gluten-free bread that is not highly processed.
13- For baking, purchase gluten-free flours such as almond flour.
14- Purchase fruits and vegetables that you can tolerate well.
15- For oil, purchase extra virgin olive oil. Avoid coconut oil.
16- Keep having turmeric, and cinnamon in your kitchen cabinet.
17- Avoid purchasing processed foods.
18- For sauces such as mayonnaise, try to purchase organic low fat and low sodium types. Avoid ketchup.
19- For beef, chicken, or vegetable broth, try to buy organic low sodium types.
20- Always purchase organic potatoes.
21- It is not recommended to purchase fruit juices with added sugar, and juices from concentrate. The best option for you is to make a juice from non-triggering fruits at home.
22- If you want to purchase almond butter, get the organic and smooth one.
23- To make your meals sweet, brown sugar might be a great option.
24- Maple syrup in limited amount (1 tbsp) may work for you as a sweetener option.
25- Try to purchase fresh foods instead of frozen or canned foods.
26- Read the ingredients of the snacks you may want to purchase. Make sure you can tolerate all ingredients well.
27- Fully avoid consuming products with High Fructose Corn Syrup (HFCS).

Cooking Tools

You do not necessarily need to buy any specific tools to cook for a person who needs to follow the low residue diet, but here are some tools that can help you ease the cooking process:

1- <u>Cast Iron skillet:</u> some people suggest having an iron skillet to absorb iron better.
2- <u>Blender:</u> for those who can use nuts in moderation, they need to blend them well. Having a suitable blender/mixer can help you cook well-blended meals such as soups, smoothies, nut butter, and juices.
3- <u>Juicer:</u> having a powerful juicer can help you taking the juices of fruits and vegetables. With this tool, you may have fruits or vegetables that cannot be tolerated because of having high insoluble fiber.
4- <u>Small lunch-dinner boxes:</u> it is recommended to eat smaller portions six times a day. One great idea to follow this eating style is to provide lunch, snacks, and dinners in separate boxes. For instance, you can put your lunch in two small lunch boxes instead of a big one, and eat each box in different time (e.g., with two hours of time-difference) at your workplace.
5- <u>Spiralizer:</u> to have spaghetti-like zucchini, potatoes, and pumpkin, you may need to have a spiralizer.
6- <u>Air fryer:</u> air frying can be a great cooking option, as it does not need much oil. You can make great zucchini or potato chip snacks or other meals using an air fryer.
7- <u>Timer and thermometer:</u> both are helpful tools for you to cook delicious meals. Remember that meats should be cooked well. Hence, you can use these tools to check if inside meats cooked well or not.

Kitchen Preparation

Here are some of the tips to prepare the kitchen and yourself before cooking:

1. Wash your hands perfectly when you want to cook.
2. Always wash fruits and vegetables before using them.
3. Remember to use allowed skin-removed or poached fruits.
4. Remember not to consume fruit cores or vegetable seeds a lot.
5. Wash meats before cooking. Use disposable gloves when washing meats and put gloves in the garbage after. Always wash your hands with warm water right after washing meats and poultries.
6. Use a separate cutting board for raw meat
7. Keep raw meats away from other foods in the kitchen and fridge.
8. Never mix cooked foods with raw meats. Mixing can happen in plates, cutting boards, etc. Never eat such foods.
9. Remember to cook or boil meats, seafood, and vegetables in perfection.
10. Keep the kitchen area well-cleaned and sanitized.

Meal Planning

1- Use proper cooking methods explained in this book. Keep your cooking style simple:
   a. If you are in remission (it seems that your symptoms are gone for couple of weeks), you are free to apply cooking techniques such as stir-fry foods in moderation with extra virgin olive oil.

b. If you are in a flare, try to stick to techniques such as boiling, steaming, and poaching.
   c. Grating spices such as ginseng is better than consuming ginseng powders.
2- You should have your meal plans ready. Use the information on this book to create your meal plans. The plans should include only foods that you can consume.
3- You also should know the strategy of finding triggering foods for yourself. To keep it simple, if you ate a specific food at any time and observed any symptoms such as diarrhea, cramping, gas, bloating, and abdominal pain, you might be intolerant to that particular food. If you ate a meal and you are not sure about the ingredient(s) you are intolerant inside, you have to write this meal in your journal and record your symptoms and conditions there. Then, you need to review your journal at the end of each week or two again and check if you can find any relations or common ingredient(s) between different meals you could not tolerate or not. You can visit a dietitian or a nutritionist to guide you more on how to find triggering foods.
4- Create at least two, two-week meal plans, with enough variety and stick to them according to your health condition. Your meal plan should have the following cooking/eating items:
   a. Meal-1: Breakfast
   b. Meal-2: Snack

The next chapter of this book gives excellent cooking recipes for IBD patients.

Chapter 5. Low Residue Diet Cooking Recipes

This chapter provides you with more than 130 fantastic delicious cooking recipes for IBD patients. It consists of various recipes to cook, serve, and enjoy, such as breakfasts, soups, salads, appetizers, main courses for lunch and dinner, desserts, drinks, and snacks.

Each cooking recipe starts with a brief introduction, preparation time, cooking time, total time, serving size, ingredients, instructions, cooking tips, Low residue diet-related tips, and nutrition facts. It has to be noted that the nutrition facts of the recipes in this book have been analyzed by "Verywell fit" Recipe Nutrition Calculator.

Breakfasts

Gluten-Free Fluffy Pancake

A great gluten-free pancake for those who cannot tolerate gluten. You can make this great pancake if you are lactose-intolerant, as well. Just remember to use lactose-free milk instead of kefir.

- Prep Time: 5 minutes
- Cook Time: 10 minutes
- Total Time: 15 minutes
- Serving: 4

Ingredients:

- 2 organic, free-range eggs
- 2 cups white rice flour or almond flour

- 2 cups kefir or (lactose-free milk with one tablespoon lemon juice)
- 1 teaspoon lime juice
- 1.5 tablespoon baking powder
- Salt to taste

Instructions

1. In a medium bowl, mix and whisk all ingredients.
2. Heat a large pan with extra virgin olive oil and cook both sides of pancakes until golden over medium heat.
3. Enjoy!

Cooking Tips:

- You can use maple syrup or honey with your pancakes if you can tolerate it.

Low residue diet-related Tips:

- Use lactose-free milk if you are lactose intolerant.

Nutrition Facts
Servings: 4

Amount per serving	
Calories	**402**
	% Daily Value*
Total Fat 7.3g	9%
Saturated Fat 3.5g	17%
Cholesterol 97mg	32%
Sodium 132mg	6%
Total Carbohydrate 71.2g	26%
Dietary Fiber 3.4g	12%
Total Sugars 6.3g	
Protein 11.5g	
Vitamin D 8mcg	39%
Calcium 20mg	2%
Iron 1mg	4%
Potassium 93mg	2%

BANANA AND APPLE PANCAKES

Another yummy lactose-free, gluten-free pancake for those on the low residue diet.

- Prep Time: 5 minutes
- Cook Time: 10 minutes
- Total Time: 15 minutes
- Serving: 2

Ingredients

- 1 apple, skin-removed
- 3 bananas, cubed
- 4 medium-sized organic, free-range eggs
- 2 cups almond flour
- 1 tablespoon extra virgin olive oil
- Honey or maple syrup (optional)

Instructions

1. In a medium bowl, mash and whisk apple, bananas, and eggs.
2. Heat a large pan with high-quality extra virgin olive oil, flatten your pancake and cook both sides until golden over medium heat.
3. Serve with honey if you can tolerate it. Enjoy!

Cooking Tips:

- You can use maple syrup or honey with your pancakes if you can tolerate it.
- Use 2 cups of white rice flour if you want to have another taste of a delicious pancake.

Nutrition Facts

Servings: 2

Amount per serving
Calories   **401**

	% Daily Value*
Total Fat 16.5g	21%
Saturated Fat 3.9g	20%
Cholesterol 327mg	109%
Sodium 126mg	5%
Total Carbohydrate 56.5g	21%
Dietary Fiber 7.3g	26%
Total Sugars 33.9g	
Protein 13.3g	
Vitamin D 31mcg	154%
Calcium 56mg	4%
Iron 3mg	14%
Potassium 871mg	19%

EGGS, SALMON, AND AVOCADO

This breakfast contains a great source of healthy fats and protein. A smooth, fast, and delicious breakfast recipe to cook!

- Prep Time: 5 minutes
- Cook Time: 10 minutes
- Total Time: 15 minutes
- Serving: 2

Ingredients:

- 2 scrambled eggs
- 2 oz salmon, cooked or canned
- 1 avocado
- 1 teaspoon extra virgin olive oil

Instructions

1. Heat a large pan with high-quality extra virgin olive oil, and scramble your eggs over medium heat.
2. Mix your scramble with avocado cubes and small salmon pieces. Enjoy!

Cooking Tips:

- You can also mash your avocado instead of cubing it.

Low residue diet-related Tips:

- Use boiled salmon and eggs if you are experiencing a severe flare-up.

Nutrition Facts
Servings: 2

Amount per serving	
Calories	**353**
	% Daily Value*
Total Fat 30.4g	39%
Saturated Fat 6.7g	34%
Cholesterol 182mg	61%
Sodium 107mg	5%
Total Carbohydrate 9.6g	3%
Dietary Fiber 6.7g	24%
Total Sugars 1.4g	
Protein 13.5g	
Vitamin D 44mcg	220%
Calcium 26mg	2%
Iron 2mg	9%
Potassium 677mg	14%

BAKED APPLE

For those who have IBD, cooked, and skin-removed fruits are great breakfast ingredients. You can use this recipe for cooking fruits like apple, peach, and pear.

- Prep Time: 5 minutes
- Cook Time: 40 minutes
- Total Time: 45 minutes
- Serving: 2

Ingredients

- 1 teaspoon cinnamon
- 1 teaspoon extra virgin olive oil
- 2 cups of water
- 2 tablespoons brown sugar

- 2 apples, cored

Instructions

1. In a medium/large pot, boil your apple with cinnamon, olive oil, water, and brown sugar over high heat for 40 minutes.
2. You can add more sugar for sweetness. However, it is not recommended for IBD patients to add more sugar.
3. Remove the apple skin, and then, enjoy!

Cooking Tips:

- You can use the same instruction to make baked fruits such as pear or peach.

Low residue diet-related Tips:

- Do not use brown sugar during a flare-up or if it irritates your gut. Simply use stevia (one tablespoon) instead.

Nutrition Facts

Servings: 2

Amount per serving

Calories	**173**
	% Daily Value*
Total Fat 2.7g	4%
Saturated Fat 0.3g	2%
Cholesterol 0mg	0%
Sodium 12mg	1%
Total Carbohydrate 40.6g	15%
Dietary Fiber 6g	21%
Total Sugars 32g	
Protein 0.7g	
Vitamin D 0mcg	0%
Calcium 27mg	2%
Iron 1mg	6%
Potassium 258mg	5%

Pear Oatmeal Bars

A great source of fiber for those who have IBD. This bar is gluten and lactose-free with a great taste of pear and ginger.

- Prep Time: 10 minutes
- Cook Time: 25 minutes
- Total Time: 35 minutes
- Serving: 4

Ingredients

- 4 organic pears
- ½ cup applesauce
- 1 teaspoon ground ginger
- ½ teaspoon salt
- ½ cup organic smooth almond butter
- 2 teaspoons pure vanilla extract
- 2 teaspoons ground cinnamon
- ¾ teaspoon baking powder
- ¾ cup oat flour (or gluten-free flour)
- ½ cup rolled oats (or a small package of ready oatmeal)

Instructions

1. Preheat oven to 375 °F.
2. Cook the pear or use a pear compote. Blend your pears to make a puree.
3. Mix your pear puree with applesauce, salt, almond butter, ginger, vanilla extract, cinnamon, baking powder, flour, and oats.
4. Pour your mix into a suitable oven pan.
5. Bake your oatmeal for 25 minutes until inside cooks well. Cut the baked oatmeal like bars.
6. Let it be cooled first and then serve!

Cooking Tips:

- It is recommended to use organic oats or ready oatmeal.
- To check if the inside cooks well, insert a toothpick inside. If it comes out without sticking to your bar, it shows that it cooked well.

Low residue diet-related Tips:

- Cook your pear or use pear compote if you cannot tolerate raw pear.
- If you have colon strictures, reduce your monthly oatmeal intakes.

Nutrition Facts
Servings: 4

Amount per serving	
Calories	**612**
	% Daily Value*
Total Fat 34.2g	44%
Saturated Fat 3.4g	17%
Cholesterol 0mg	0%
Sodium 296mg	13%
Total Carbohydrate 70g	25%
Dietary Fiber 18.2g	65%
Total Sugars 27.9g	
Protein 14.5g	
Vitamin D 0mcg	0%
Calcium 249mg	19%
Iron 4mg	23%
Potassium 931mg	20%

Avocado & Egg Breakfast Toast

A very simple, delicious breakfast dish, high in protein and healthy fat.

- Prep Time: 5 minutes
- Cook Time: 10 minutes
- Total Time: 15 minutes
- Serving: 2

Ingredients

- 4 slices of white toast or gluten-free bread
- ½ cup low fat cottage cheese or lactose-free Havarti cheese
- 1 avocado
- 2 large organic free-range eggs
- 4 egg whites
- 1 tablespoon lime juice
- Salt and pepper to taste

Instructions

1. Toast your white bread toasts the way you want.
2. Mix cheese, eggs, egg whites, salt, and pepper in a bowl and scramble it in a pan over medium heat for 7 minutes.
3. Coat your toasts with scrambled mix and mashed avocado. Then, squeeze lime. Enjoy!

Cooking Tips:

- You can use low-fat feta cheese instead of cottage cheese, as well.

Low residue diet-related Tips:

- Boil your eggs if you are experiencing a severe flare-up.
- Do not use black pepper if you are in a flare-up.

Nutrition Facts	
Servings: 2	
Amount per serving	
Calories	**411**
	% Daily Value*
Total Fat 26.4g	34%
Saturated Fat 6.5g	32%
Cholesterol 191mg	64%
Sodium 467mg	20%
Total Carbohydrate 21.2g	8%
Dietary Fiber 7.2g	26%
Total Sugars 2.5g	
Protein 24.7g	
Vitamin D 18mcg	88%
Calcium 103mg	8%
Iron 2mg	12%
Potassium 751mg	16%

SMOOTHIE BOWL

A mix of skin-removed and chopped fruits can create a tremendous rich breakfast!

- Prep Time: 10 minutes
- Cook Time: 0 minutes
- Total Time: 10 minutes
- Serving: 2

Ingredients

- 1 banana, sliced
- 1 cup almond milk or lactose-free milk
- 1 cup papaya chunks
- 1 cup diced mango

Instructions

1. Blend all mentioned ingredients in a blender. Serve and Enjoy!

Cooking Tips:

- You can use the same instruction to make fruit bowls with other fruits you can tolerate.

- You can add 1 cup of papaya to your bowl as well.

Low residue diet-related Tips:

- Use ¼ mango if you are experiencing a severe flare-up or, instead, use 1 cup of papaya.

Nutrition Facts	
Servings: 2	
Amount per serving	
Calories	419
	% Daily Value*
Total Fat 29.2g	37%
Saturated Fat 25.5g	128%
Cholesterol 0mg	0%
Sodium 20mg	1%
Total Carbohydrate 43.3g	16%
Dietary Fiber 6.6g	24%
Total Sugars 30.6g	
Protein 4.5g	
Vitamin D 0mcg	0%
Calcium 42mg	3%
Iron 2mg	14%
Potassium 755mg	16%

Zucchini Bread Oatmeal

Enjoy the taste of grated zucchini and oatmeal and have a healthy breakfast!

- Prep Time: 5 minutes
- Cook Time: 7 minutes
- Total Time: 12 minutes
- Serving: 2

Ingredients

- ⅓ cup organic rolled oats or ready oatmeal
- 1 cup unsweetened almond or lactose-free milk
- ½ teaspoon cinnamon powder
- ½ cup zucchini
- 1 teaspoon vanilla extract
- Maple syrup (optional)

Instructions

1. Mix your milk with cinnamon and oat in a medium pot and boil the mixture over medium heat for 4 minutes.
2. Grate zucchini, add it to the mix, and stir well for three minutes.
3. In a small bowl, mix vanilla extract and maple syrup.
4. When oatmeal cooked, remove from heat and pour the syrup on it.
5. Let it be cooled and then serve!

Cooking Tips:

- You can use maple or agave syrup in this recipe if you can tolerate it.

Low residue diet-related Tips:

- If you have colon strictures due to IBD, reduce your monthly oatmeal intakes. Avoid any types of seeds.

Nutrition Facts
Servings: 2

Amount per serving	
Calories	**82**
	% Daily Value*
Total Fat 2.7g	3%
Saturated Fat 0.3g	2%
Cholesterol 0mg	0%
Sodium 94mg	4%
Total Carbohydrate 11.5g	4%
Dietary Fiber 2.2g	8%
Total Sugars 0.9g	
Protein 2.6g	
Vitamin D 1mcg	3%
Calcium 162mg	12%
Iron 1mg	6%
Potassium 222mg	5%

BREAKFAST FRUIT SALAD

A mix of a variety of fruits (skin-removed and chopped) can create an excellent breakfast salad for IBD patients!

- Prep Time: 5 minutes
- Cook Time: 25 minutes
- Total Time: 30 minutes
- Serving: 6

Ingredients

- 2 large firm bananas, cubed
- 1 medium mango, skin removed and cubed
- 1 medium green apple, skin removed and cubed
- 1 medium papaya, skin-removed and cubed
- 1 tablespoon lemon juice
- ½ cup sugar or 1 tablespoon stevia (optional)
- ⅓ cup orange juice (optional)

Instructions

1. Mix all fruits in a bowl.
2. Boil your orange juice, lemon juice, and sugar in a small pot (over high heat). Stir well.
3. Let the juice be cooled. Then, add your cooled juice to the fruit bowl. Enjoy!

Cooking Tips:

- You can use orange juice in this recipe if you can tolerate it.

Low residue diet-related Tips:

- If you are experiencing a severe flare-up, cook your fruits first.

Nutrition Facts	
Servings: 6	
Amount per serving	
Calories	**108**
	% Daily Value*
Total Fat 0.4g	1%
Saturated Fat 0.1g	1%
Cholesterol 0mg	0%
Sodium 6mg	0%
Total Carbohydrate 27.7g	10%
Dietary Fiber 3.5g	13%
Total Sugars 18.8g	
Protein 1g	
Vitamin D 0mcg	0%
Calcium 17mg	1%
Iron 1mg	3%
Potassium 331mg	7%

Banana Split Oatmeal

A great combination of oatmeal and banana can make a great breakfast full of fiber and potassium.

- Prep Time: 10 minutes
- Cook Time: 0 minutes
- Total Time: 10 minutes
- Serving: 2

Ingredients

- ½ cup water, almond milk or lactose-free milk
- 1 cup old-fashioned rolled oats or a small ready oatmeal package
- ½ banana, cubed
- Salt to taste

Instructions

1. Boil your milk or water in a pot over high heat.
2. Add oat and salt to it. Stir for two more minutes.
3. Serve your oatmeal with cubed bananas. Enjoy!

Cooking Tips:

- You can use honey, maple or agave syrup in this recipe if you can tolerate.

Low residue diet-related Tips:

- If you have colon strictures due to IBD, reduce your monthly oatmeal intakes.

Nutrition Facts	
Servings: 2	
Amount per serving	
Calories	**319**
	% Daily Value*
Total Fat 17.1g	22%
Saturated Fat 13.2g	66%
Cholesterol 0mg	0%
Sodium 89mg	4%
Total Carbohydrate 37.8g	14%
Dietary Fiber 8.2g	22%
Total Sugars 6g	
Protein 7.1g	
Vitamin D 0mcg	0%
Calcium 32mg	2%
Iron 3mg	16%
Potassium 412mg	9%

EGG TACOS WITH AVOCADO

Enjoy a breakfast sandwich with egg and avocado, which is full of healthy fats and functional proteins.

- Prep Time: 5 minutes
- Cook Time: 10 minutes
- Total Time: 15 minutes
- Serving: 2

Ingredients

- 4 small tortillas
- 2 organic, free-range eggs
- 1 avocado
- Salt to taste

Instructions

1. Warm or toast tortillas.
2. Scramble or boil your eggs using salt.
3. Mash your avocado
4. Fill your tortillas with avocado and eggs. Enjoy!

Cooking Tips:

- You can use white bread or gluten-free bread (if you can tolerate them) instead of tortillas.

Low residue diet-related Tips:

- If you have colon strictures or flare-up due to IBD, use very soft bread with white flour-like a white pita. If you are sensitive to gluten, use soft gluten-free white rice bread.

Nutrition Facts
Servings: 2

Amount per serving
Calories 373

	% Daily Value*
Total Fat 25.3g	32%
Saturated Fat 5.7g	29%
Cholesterol 164mg	55%
Sodium 167mg	7%
Total Carbohydrate 30.4g	11%
Dietary Fiber 9.8g	35%
Total Sugars 1.3g	
Protein 10.2g	
Vitamin D 15mcg	77%
Calcium 74mg	6%
Iron 2mg	11%
Potassium 636mg	14%

CRISPY HASH BROWN WITH EGG

Start your day with hash brown and egg! A great combination, as always!

- Prep Time: 20 minutes
- Cook Time: 15 minutes
- Total Time: 35 minutes

- Serving: 2

Ingredients

- 2 large yellow potatoes, shredded
- ¼ cup all-purpose flour or gluten-free flour
- 2 tablespoons extra virgin olive oil
- 2 organic range-free eggs
- Salt and pepper to taste

Instructions

1. Shred potatoes and rinse them until the water cleared. Dry potatoes.
2. Mix your potatoes with flour, eggs, salt, and pepper.
3. Flatten your mix in a large skillet and let it cook over medium heat until golden brown. Flip and cook the other side.
4. Remove from the skillet and drain with a paper towel. Enjoy!

Cooking Tips:

- To flip it quickly, you can cut in half or quarter.

Low residue diet-related Tips:

- Do not use pepper if you are experiencing a severe flare-up. Try to boil and mash your potatoes as well.

Nutrition Facts	
Servings: 2	
Amount per serving	
Calories	**385**
	% Daily Value*
Total Fat 18.7g	24%
Saturated Fat 3.4g	17%
Cholesterol 164mg	55%
Sodium 70mg	3%
Total Carbohydrate 45.9g	17%
Dietary Fiber 2.8g	10%
Total Sugars 3g	
Protein 10.2g	
Vitamin D 15mcg	77%
Calcium 34mg	3%
Iron 2mg	12%
Potassium 686mg	15%

GRILLED ALMOND BUTTER HONEY BANANA SANDWICH

An excellent easy to make a sandwich for your breakfast.

- Prep Time: 5 minutes
- Cook Time: 0 minutes
- Total Time: 5 minutes
- Serving: 2

Ingredients

- 1 tablespoon extra virgin olive oil
- Few grams of almond butter
- 1 banana
- 4 slices of white bread or gluten-free bread
- Honey or maple syrup to taste

Instructions

- Toast your bread slices, as you desired.
- Mash banana, coat your bread with banana, almond butter, and honey (maple syrup). Enjoy!

Cooking Tips:

- You can use honey, maple or agave syrup in this recipe if you can tolerate.

Low residue diet-related Tips:

- If you have colon stricture(s) due to IBD, make sure you are using smoothened types of almond butter.

Nutrition Facts
Servings: 2

Amount per serving
Calories 172

	% Daily Value*
Total Fat 8.7g	11%
Saturated Fat 1.3g	6%
Cholesterol 0mg	0%
Sodium 123mg	5%
Total Carbohydrate 23.3g	8%
Dietary Fiber 2.1g	8%
Total Sugars 8.4g	
Protein 2.4g	
Vitamin D 0mcg	0%
Calcium 31mg	2%
Iron 1mg	6%
Potassium 241mg	5%

Avocado-Cheese Bagel

If you are in love with a bagel, you will enjoy making an avocado-cheese bagel recipe.

- Prep Time: 5 minutes
- Cook Time: 0 minutes
- Total Time: 5 minutes
- Serving: 1

Ingredients

- 1 white bagel or gluten-free bread, toasted
- 2 tablespoons low-fat feta cheese or lactose-free Swiss cheese
- ½ avocado, mashed
- Salt to taste

Instructions

- Open the bagel and coat a half with cheese, avocado (mashed), and salt.
- Cover with the other half. Enjoy!

Cooking Tips:

- Use bagels with white flour.
- You may want to add fresh lemon juice to your avocado for another great taste and avoid turning avocado to brown.

Low residue diet-related Tips:

- If you have colon strictures due to IBD, make sure you are using seedless bagels.

Nutrition Facts	
Servings: 1	
Amount per serving	
Calories	525
	% Daily Value*
Total Fat 21.3g	27%
Saturated Fat 4.4g	22%
Cholesterol 3mg	1%
Sodium 896mg	39%
Total Carbohydrate 66.2g	24%
Dietary Fiber 9.3g	33%
Total Sugars 6.3g	
Protein 19.9g	
Vitamin D 0mcg	0%
Calcium 210mg	16%
Iron 5mg	28%
Potassium 572mg	12%

Apple Cinnamon Oatmeal

Enjoy tasting a traditional apple cinnamon oatmeal that can be prepared in less than 15 minutes.

- Prep Time: 5 minutes
- Cook Time: 15 minutes
- Total Time: 20 minutes

- Serving: 2

Ingredients

- 1 tablespoon extra virgin olive oil
- 1 cup gluten-free ground oats or ready oatmeal
- 2 cups unsweetened almond or lactose-free milk
- ½ teaspoon cinnamon
- 1 large apple, sliced and skin-removed
- 1 tablespoon maple syrup, or agave syrup
- ¼ cup pomegranate juice (optional)

Instructions

- Preheat oven to 375 °F.
- In a medium bowl, mix and whisk oats with cinnamon, oil, apple, pomegranate juice (optional), maple syrup, and milk.
- Use a suitable baking pan or sheet. Spread your mix to it and bake for 15 minutes until golden brown.

Cooking Tips:

- You can prepare this breakfast in a large skillet over medium heat for 10-15 minutes until brown.
- Use agave syrup or 1 teaspoon of stevia if you cannot tolerate maple syrup or honey.

Low residue diet-related Tips:

- If you have colon strictures due to IBD, make sure you are using less oatmeal monthly.
- Use pomegranate juice only if you can tolerate it.
- If you are experiencing a flare-up, cook your apple first.

Nutrition Facts	
Servings: 2	
Amount per serving	
Calories	**276**
	% Daily Value*
Total Fat 12.5g	16%
Saturated Fat 1.3g	7%
Cholesterol 0mg	0%
Sodium 182mg	8%
Total Carbohydrate 40.6g	15%
Dietary Fiber 6.5g	23%
Total Sugars 17.6g	
Protein 4.8g	
Vitamin D 1mcg	7%
Calcium 323mg	25%
Iron 3mg	15%
Potassium 332mg	7%

APPETIZERS

Turkey Potpie Soup

Great soup with perfect ingredients for IBD patients.

- Prep Time: 10 minutes
- Cook Time: 35 minutes
- Total Time: 45 minutes
- Serving: 4

Ingredients

- ¼ cup white gluten-free flour or refined all-purpose flour
- 16 oz turkey breast, cubed
- 2 cups turkey/chicken stock, divided
- 4 cups fat-free milk or lactose-free cow milk
- 1 teaspoon turmeric powder
- 2 celery stalks, chopped in small pieces
- 1 large carrot, cubed 1 inch (~2.54 cm)
- 2 medium potatoes, peeled and cubed 1 inch (~2.54 cm)
- Salt and pepper, to taste

Instructions

1. Mix 1 cup of turkey/chicken broth with flour and whisk well. Set aside.
2. Pour another cup of broth into a large pot. Add turkey, celery, potatoes and turmeric powder inside and boil until vegetables and turkey get soft.
3. Warm milk and add to the mix. Then, add carrots and cook for another 5 minutes. Add salt and pepper to taste.

Cooking Tips:

- You may want to add one cup of mushroom if you can tolerate it.
- You can remove flour from the recipe if you do not have one or do not want a soup with a thick texture.
- You can make this soup with chicken breasts as well.

Low residue diet-related Tips:

- If you cannot tolerate ordinary mushrooms, you may try Shiitake mushroom.
- Do not use pepper if you are experiencing a severe flare-up.

Nutrition Facts	
Servings: 4	
Amount per serving	
Calories	**326**
	% Daily Value*
Total Fat 2.4g	3%
Saturated Fat 0.5g	3%
Cholesterol 54mg	18%
Sodium 1696mg	74%
Total Carbohydrate 42.3g	15%
Dietary Fiber 4.2g	15%
Total Sugars 18.6g	
Protein 30.8g	
Vitamin D 1mcg	6%
Calcium 341mg	26%
Iron 3mg	16%
Potassium 1286mg	27%

POTATO-GINGER MISO SOUP

A fabulous Miso soup with GI healing ingredients. A great source of required vitamins and minerals for IBD patients:

- Prep Time: 10 minutes
- Cook Time: 30 minutes
- Total Time: 40 minutes
- Serving: 3-4

Ingredients

- 1 fresh ginger or ½ tablespoon fresh grated ginger
- 2 cups sodium-free/low sodium vegetable broth
- 2 tablespoons miso
- 2 medium potatoes, peeled and cubed 1 inch (~2.54 cm)
- ½ cup unsweetened almond milk
- ½ teaspoon salt

Instructions

1. Boil potatoes in a medium pot until softened.
2. Drain and mash your potatoes.

3. In a medium/large pot, mix broth, ginger, and salt, and boil over medium heat.
4. Add mashed potatoes to the mix and blend until smoothened.
5. Add warm miso and almond milk. Blend again until smoothened. Then, heat the soup for 5 more minutes over medium heat. Enjoy!

Cooking Tips:

- You can add 1 cup of chicken breast to the recipe if you want to have chicken miso.

Nutrition Facts

Servings: 3

Amount per serving

Calories	**242**
	% Daily Value*
Total Fat 11.3g	15%
Saturated Fat 8.9g	45%
Cholesterol 0mg	0%
Sodium 951mg	41%
Total Carbohydrate 28.8g	10%
Dietary Fiber 5g	18%
Total Sugars 4.2g	
Protein 8g	
Vitamin D 0mcg	0%
Calcium 33mg	3%
Iron 2mg	12%
Potassium 857mg	18%

Parsnip/Carrot Potato Soup

The parsnip is a root vegetable from the carrot family. Do not use parsnip if you are in a flare-up. Instead, use carrot in the recipe.

- Prep Time: 10 minutes
- Cook Time: 30 minutes
- Total Time: 40 minutes
- Serving: 4

Ingredients

- 1 celery stalk, chopped
- 4 parsnips or carrots, cubed 1 inch (~2.54 cm)
- 3 cups chicken broth
- 1 tablespoon extra virgin olive oil
- 2 potatoes, skin removed and cubed 1 inch (~2.54 cm)
- 1 teaspoon salt
- 2 tablespoons low-fat feta cheese or lactose-free Havarti cheese (optional)
- 1 teaspoon pepper (optional)

Instructions

6. Choose a large pan and cook celery and parsnip (carrot) using extra virgin olive oil over medium heat and occasionally mix until semi-soft texture.
7. Warm up the broth and pour it into the pan. Add potato, salt, and pepper (optional) and cook for 20 minutes.
8. Enjoy the soup as it is or blend it for having a puree.
9. Sprinkle low-fat feta cheese or lactose-free Havarti cheese on top if you desire.

Cooking Tips:

- You can mix all ingredients at the same time and let it boil for 25-30 minutes.

Low residue diet-related Tips:

- Do not use parsnip if you cannot tolerate it, or you are experiencing a severe flare-up. Instead, use carrots.

- Do not use pepper if you are experiencing a severe flare-up.

Nutrition Facts
Servings: 4

Amount per serving	
Calories	**184**
	% Daily Value*
Total Fat 4.9g	6%
Saturated Fat 0.9g	4%
Cholesterol 0mg	0%
Sodium 593mg	26%
Total Carbohydrate 29.7g	11%
Dietary Fiber 6g	21%
Total Sugars 5.1g	
Protein 6.3g	
Vitamin D 0mcg	0%
Calcium 45mg	3%
Iron 1mg	7%
Potassium 864mg	18%

Pumpkin Soup

Great semi-classical pumpkin soup can be one of your choices to make every week.

- Prep Time: 15 minutes
- Cook Time: 15 minutes
- Total Time: 30 minutes
- Serving: 4-6

Ingredients

- 2 lbs (~1 kg) pumpkin, skin-removed, seeds-removed, chopped
- 1 large carrot, skin-removed, diced
- 2 large potatoes, skin removed, diced
- 4 cups sodium-free/low sodium chicken broth
- ½ cup milk or lactose-free cow milk
- Salt and pepper, to taste
- 2 chicken bouillon cubes (optional)

Instructions

1. Mix and boil all ingredients in a large pot over medium heat.
2. Remove from heat. Blend the soup until smooth.
3. Add salt, and pepper to taste

Cooking Tips:

- If you can tolerate and if you can find a very light cream/sour cream, you can use it instead of milk.
- If you are in remission, you can cook vegetables first in a large skillet by 1 tablespoon extra virgin olive oil over medium heat until semi-soft texture. Then, boil and blend.

Low residue diet-related Tips:

- Do not use pepper if you are experiencing a severe flare-up.

Nutrition Facts
Servings: 6

Amount per serving	
Calories	**174**
	% Daily Value*
Total Fat 1.5g	2%
Saturated Fat 0.5g	3%
Cholesterol 0mg	0%
Sodium 543mg	24%
Total Carbohydrate 34.3g	12%
Dietary Fiber 7.6g	27%
Total Sugars 8.5g	
Protein 7.8g	
Vitamin D 0mcg	1%
Calcium 86mg	7%
Iron 3mg	17%
Potassium 988mg	21%

Stracciatella Soup

This delicious Italian soup is entirely in line with patient tolerance levels full of healthy ingredients. It can significantly supply your protein.

- Prep Time: 10 minutes
- Cook Time: 15 minutes
- Total Time: 25 minutes
- Serving: 4

Ingredients

- 6 cups low sodium/sodium-free chicken broth
- 2 tablespoons semolina flour or all-purpose gluten-free flour
- 3 large organic free-range eggs
- Salt and pepper, to taste
- 1 tablespoon hard pecorino cheese, grated
- 1 tablespoon hard Parmigiano-Reggiano cheese, grated
- 1 tablespoon fresh parsley (optional)

Instructions

1. In a large pot and over high heat, bring chicken stock to simmer. Add salt and pepper.
2. In a large bowl, whisk eggs, semolina or all-purpose gluten-free flour, Parmigiano-Reggiano, and pecorino cheese altogether.
3. Slowly pour the egg mixture into your pot and simmer well. Let the soup simmer.
4. Serve and garnish it with parsley if you want. Enjoy!

Cooking Tips:

- Most aged cheddar-type cheese is lactose-free. As such, lactose-intolerant patients can tolerate pecorino and Parmigiano-Reggiano. However, they should be used in moderation during a flare-up.

Low residue diet-related Tips:

- Use pecorino and Parmigiano-Reggiano in moderation if you are in a flare-up or simply remove them from the recipe.
- Do not use pepper if you are experiencing a severe flare-up.

Nutrition Facts
Servings: 4

Amount per serving
Calories 164

	% Daily Value*
Total Fat 8.3g	11%
Saturated Fat 3.5g	18%
Cholesterol 147mg	49%
Sodium 1277mg	56%
Total Carbohydrate 5.5g	2%
Dietary Fiber 0.2g	1%
Total Sugars 1.3g	
Protein 15.4g	
Vitamin D 13mcg	66%
Calcium 120mg	9%
Iron 2mg	9%
Potassium 376mg	8%

HAM AND POTATO SOUP

A delicious soup for IBD patients who love ham.

- Prep Time: 10 minutes
- Cook Time: 20 minutes
- Total Time: 30 minutes
- Serving: 4

Ingredients

- 2 large potatoes, peeled and cubed 1 inch (~2.54 cm)
- 1 cup cooked ham, diced and cubed 1 inch (~2.54 cm)
- 3 cups sodium-free/low sodium chicken broth
- 1 tablespoon extra virgin olive oil

- ¼ cup white all-purpose flour or gluten-free flour
- ½ cup celery stalk, diced
- 2 cups milk, or lactose-free cow milk
- Salt and pepper to taste

Instructions

1. Boil potatoes, celery, ham, and chicken broth in a large pot over medium heat for 15 minutes.
2. In a large pan, pour high-quality extra virgin olive oil and whisk flour over medium heat. Stir consistently until golden brown. Warm milk and add slowly to the flour. Stir continuously for five minutes.
3. Pour the mix into the pot and stir. Add salt and pepper to taste. Enjoy!

Cooking Tips:

- For having a classic taste, you can use honey ham.

Low residue diet-related Tips:

- If you are in a severe flare-up, avoid using ham/honey ham. Instead, use fat-removed pork tenderloin or chicken breasts.
- Do not use pepper if you are experiencing a severe flare-up.

Nutrition Facts
Servings: 4

Amount per serving	
Calories	**316**
	% Daily Value*
Total Fat 9.2g	12%
Saturated Fat 3.1g	15%
Cholesterol 29mg	10%
Sodium 935mg	41%
Total Carbohydrate 43.3g	16%
Dietary Fiber 5.3g	19%
Total Sugars 8.2g	
Protein 16.1g	
Vitamin D 1mcg	3%
Calcium 190mg	15%
Iron 2mg	12%
Potassium 1112mg	24%

BUTTERNUT SQUASH SOUP

A perfect soup for people with IBD to be included in their weekly diet.

- Prep Time: 10 minutes
- Cook Time: 55 minutes
- Total Time: 65 minutes
- Serving: 6

Ingredients

- 3 lbs (~1.5 kg) butternut squash, halved & skin-removed
- 2 carrots, peeled and cubed
- 3-4 cups low sodium chicken or vegetable stock/broth
- 2 chicken or beef bouillon cubes
- ¼ cup olive oil (for roasting option)
- 2 teaspoons salt, to taste
- 1 teaspoon ground black pepper, to taste (optional)

Instructions

1. Boil all ingredients in a large pot over medium heat for 40 minutes until softened. Remove from the pot. Allow to cool down for 5-10 minutes.
2. Pour all ingredients into a blender. Then, blend until smooth. Serve hot and enjoy!

Cooking Tips:

- For having a classic taste, you can use low-fat cream/sour cream on top if you can tolerate it.
- Be careful with the steam that may come out of the blended soup.

Nutrition Facts
Servings: 6

Amount per serving	
Calories	**193**
	% Daily Value*
Total Fat 8.7g	11%
Saturated Fat 1.3g	7%
Cholesterol 0mg	0%
Sodium 1037mg	45%
Total Carbohydrate 29.3g	11%
Dietary Fiber 5g	18%
Total Sugars 6.2g	
Protein 3.6g	
Vitamin D 0mcg	0%
Calcium 117mg	9%
Iron 2mg	10%
Potassium 869mg	18%

CHICKEN NOODLE SOUP

The chicken noodle soup is one of the famed soups all around the world. Enjoy making it in less than 45 minutes!

- Prep Time: 5 minutes
- Cook Time: 40 minutes
- Total Time: 45 minutes
- Serving: 6

Ingredients

- 1 cup vermicelli or egg noodles or rice noodles (gluten-free option)
- 8 skin-removed chicken legs
- 1-2 chicken bouillon cube(s), crushed
- 2 cups of water
- 1 tablespoon extra virgin olive oil
- 2 teaspoons salt, to taste
- 2 large carrots, cubed & skin-removed
- 1 celery stalk, chopped
- 6 cups low sodium chicken stock/broth
- 1 teaspoon ground black pepper, to taste (optional)
- ¼ cup fresh parsley, chopped (optional)

Instructions

1. In a large skillet, heat high-quality olive oil over medium heat and cook celery and carrots for 5 minutes.
2. Pour chicken broth into the skillet, add and cook chicken legs.
3. Add crushed bouillons and water to cover all ingredients.
4. When chicken cooked, use a plate to shred it and remove the bone.
5. Bring shredded chickens back to the soup and add noodles. Add salt, and pepper. Cover it for 7 minutes. Then, open the lid and stir well.
6. Serve in a bowl and garnish with chopped fresh parsley (optional)

Cooking Tips:

- You can use skin-removed chicken thighs or breasts instead of chicken legs, as well.

- You can use gluten-free noodles if you are gluten-intolerant.

Nutrition Facts	
Servings: 6	
Amount per serving	
Calories	**420**
	% Daily Value*
Total Fat 13.9g	18%
Saturated Fat 3.3g	17%
Cholesterol 120mg	40%
Sodium 1175mg	51%
Total Carbohydrate 28.3g	10%
Dietary Fiber 1.8g	6%
Total Sugars 3.2g	
Protein 41.9g	
Vitamin D 0mcg	0%
Calcium 27mg	2%
Iron 3mg	19%
Potassium 348mg	7%

CREAMY CHICKEN SOUP

A very delicious savory soup specially modified for IBD patients.

- Prep Time: 5 minutes
- Cook Time: 30 minutes
- Total Time: 35 minutes
- Serving: 4-6

Ingredients

- 1.5 lbs boneless, skin-removed chicken breast
- 1 cup carrots, skin-removed and cubed 1 inch (~2.54 cm)
- 1 medium potato, skin-removed and cubed 1 inch (~2.54 cm)
- 2 tablespoons extra virgin olive oil
- 1 cup low-fat milk or lactose-free cow milk
- 3 cups low-sodium chicken broth
- 1 teaspoon turmeric powder

- Salt and pepper, to taste
- ½ teaspoon dried thyme
- 1-2 tablespoon(s) lemon juice
- 1 cup mushrooms (optional)
- 1 cup cream/sour cream (optional)

Instructions

1. Heat extra virgin olive oil in a large pot and cook chicken over medium heat with turmeric, salt, and pepper until golden brown both sides. Remove chickens.
2. Add carrots, potato, thyme, and mushroom (optional) to the pot. Stir well until half-cooked. Add chicken broth. Then, let it cook for 15-20 minutes.
3. Add warm milk and 1-2 tablespoon(s) lemon juice. Let it simmer for five more minutes. Serve warm and enjoy!

Cooking Tips:

- You can use ½ cup shiitake mushroom if regular mushrooms irritate your gut, or remove mushroom from the recipe.
- You can add sour cream on top of the soup if you can tolerate it during remissions.

Low residue diet-related Tips:

- Do not use pepper if you are experiencing a severe flare-up.
- If you are in extreme flare-up condition, boil chicken as well.

Nutrition Facts
Servings: 6

Amount per serving
Calories 224

	% Daily Value*
Total Fat 6.7g	9%
Saturated Fat 1g	5%
Cholesterol 68mg	23%
Sodium 145mg	6%
Total Carbohydrate 10.9g	4%
Dietary Fiber 1.4g	5%
Total Sugars 3.4g	
Protein 29.6g	
Vitamin D 21mcg	106%
Calcium 61mg	5%
Iron 2mg	8%
Potassium 285mg	6%

S*eafood* C*howder* S*oup*

A must-try recipe if you are in love with seafood!

- Prep Time: 10 minutes
- Cook Time: 25 minutes
- Total Time: 35 minutes
- Serving: 4-6

Ingredients

- 3 potatoes, peeled and cubed 1 inch (~2.54 cm)
- 2 cups of low-sodium vegetable broth or chicken broth
- ¾ cup of milk, or lactose-free cow milk
- 4 oz salmon filet, peeled and cubed
- 4 oz codfish filet, peeled and cubed
- 8 raw shrimps, peeled
- 2 tablespoons fresh lemon juice
- 1 bay leaf
- ½ teaspoon grated ginger
- Salt and pepper to taste

Instructions

1. In a large pot, warm chicken broth and add potatoes, bay leaf, salmon, and cod.
2. Let the soup cook for 15 minutes over medium heat. Stir occasionally. Cover but leave a corner open for the steam to escape.
3. Add warm milk, shrimp, lemon juice, ginger, sale, and pepper to the soup. Stir for 5-10 minutes. Enjoy!

Cooking Tips:

- You can add ⅓ cup of crab into the soup if you like.
- You can add sour cream on top of the soup if you can tolerate it.

Low residue diet-related Tips:

- Do not use pepper if you are experiencing a severe flare-up.

Nutrition Facts
Servings: 6

Amount per serving	
Calories	**268**
	% Daily Value*
Total Fat 7.1g	9%
Saturated Fat 1.6g	8%
Cholesterol 134mg	45%
Sodium 285mg	12%
Total Carbohydrate 20.5g	7%
Dietary Fiber 3g	11%
Total Sugars 3.7g	
Protein 31.4g	
Vitamin D 0mcg	1%
Calcium 112mg	9%
Iron 2mg	10%
Potassium 772mg	16%

Barley/Oatmeal Soup

A delicious Mediterranean soup with healthy, rich ingredients for IBD patients!

- Prep Time: 10 minutes

- Soak Time: 120 minutes
- Cook Time: 40 minutes
- Total Time: 50 (or 170) minutes
- Serving: 6

Ingredients

- 1 cup barley or oatmeal
- 1 tablespoon all-purpose white flour or gluten-free flour
- 1.5 cup low-fat milk or lactose-free cow milk
- 1 cup carrot, peeled and cubed 1 inch (~2.54 cm)
- 7 cups low-sodium chicken broth
- 1 tablespoon extra virgin olive oil
- 1 tablespoon fresh lemon, squeezed
- Salt & pepper, to taste
- 1 tablespoon parsley, chopped (optional)

Instructions

1. First, let the barley soak for 2 hours. You can use oatmeal if you do not want to wait for 2 hours.
2. In a large pot, cook barley (or oatmeal) and carrots with chicken broth over medium heat for 30 minutes. Add salt and pepper. Stir occasionally.
3. In a medium pan, make a béchamel sauce: heat extra virgin olive oil. Add flour to the oil and stir until golden brown. Slowly add warm milk to the pan and stir perfectly until thickened. If the sauce is very thick, add more milk.
4. Add béchamel sauce to the pot and add lemon juice. Stir well over low heat for 5-10 more minutes.
5. Garnish the top with chopped parsley. Enjoy!

Cooking Tips:

- You may want to add ½ cup skin-removed chicken breast to your soup to make a chicken-barley soup.
- An orange-color barley soup can be made by one tablespoon tomato paste and 1 cup of water instead of 1.5 cups of milk.

Low residue diet-related Tips:

- Do not use pepper and parsley if you are experiencing a severe flare-up.
- If you cannot tolerate tomato, do not use the orange version of this soup explained in the cooking tips section.

Nutrition Facts
Servings: 6

Amount per serving	
Calories	**185**
	% Daily Value*
Total Fat 3.7g	5%
Saturated Fat 0.9g	4%
Cholesterol 3mg	1%
Sodium 125mg	5%
Total Carbohydrate 29.8g	11%
Dietary Fiber 5.9g	21%
Total Sugars 4.4g	
Protein 8.5g	
Vitamin D 32mcg	159%
Calcium 89mg	7%
Iron 2mg	9%
Potassium 293mg	6%

Homemade Vegetable Broth

It is an excellent idea for people living with IBD to make their homemade vegetable broth instead of purchasing it from the stores. Many vegetable products are high in sodium and are mixed vegetables that cannot be well-tolerated by IBD patients.

- Prep Time: 10 minutes
- Cook Time: 45 minutes
- Total Time: 55 minutes

- Serving: 4-6

Ingredients

- 4 cups celery, chopped
- 4 cups carrot, skin-removed and cubed
- 4 cups of water
- 2 tablespoons fresh lemon juice
- 2 tablespoons extra virgin olive oil
- ½ tablespoon turmeric powder
- 1 bay leaf
- ½ tablespoon salt, to taste
- 1 tablespoon fresh parsley, chopped (optional)
- ½ teaspoon pepper (optional)

Instructions

1. Choose a large pan and cook vegetables with extra virgin olive oil, turmeric powder, salt, and pepper over medium heat until golden brown.
2. Put ingredients in the pan into a large pot, add water, lemon juice, bay leaf, and chopped fresh parsley (optional). Thoroughly boil over low heat until all ingredients get soft.
3. Clear the broth by a colander. Serve immediately or pour and store in a suitable bottle for further use.

Cooking Tips:

- You can blend all ingredients to have a smoothened soup instead of broth.

Low residue diet-related Tips:

- Do not use pepper, and fresh parsley if you are experiencing a severe flare-up.

Nutrition Facts	
Servings: 4	
Amount per serving	
Calories	**127**
	% Daily Value*
Total Fat 7.4g	9%
Saturated Fat 1.1g	6%
Cholesterol 0mg	0%
Sodium 1038mg	45%
Total Carbohydrate 14.9g	5%
Dietary Fiber 4.7g	17%
Total Sugars 7g	
Protein 1.8g	
Vitamin D 0mcg	0%
Calcium 90mg	7%
Iron 1mg	6%
Potassium 650mg	14%

HOMEMADE BEEF BROTH

An excellent idea for people living with IBD to make their homemade beef broth instead of purchasing it from the stores. Many vegetable products are high in sodium and fat that are not good for IBD patients. Beef broth is an excellent option for IBD patients to consume when they are experiencing a flare-up.

- Prep Time: 10 minutes
- Cook Time: 60 minutes
- Total Time: 70 minutes
- Serving: 4-6

Ingredients

- 6 lbs organic grass-fed beef bones
- 2 celery stalks, chopped
- 3 carrots, chopped
- 3 bay leaves
- 1 teaspoon turmeric
- 1 tablespoon extra virgin olive oil
- 1 teaspoon dried thyme
- 2 tablespoons salt

- 1 teaspoon black pepper (optional)

Instructions

1. Preheat oven to 400 °F.
2. Roast your bones, celery, carrots with extra virgin olive oil in the oven for 40 minutes.
3. At the same time, boil water and add bay leaves, turmeric, thyme, salt and pepper to it.
4. Add the roasted bones and vegetables to the water. Water should be enough to cover all ingredients.
5. Lid ajar and simmer all mix over slow heat for 20 minutes.
6. Remove all bones.
7. Clear the broth by a colander. Serve immediately or pour and store in a suitable bottle or jar for further use.

Cooking Tips:

- You can blend all ingredients to have a smoothened soup instead of broth, especially if you cooked meat pieces with bones.

Low residue diet-related Tips:

- Do not use pepper if you are experiencing a flare-up.

Nutrition Facts	
Servings: 4	
Amount per serving	
Calories	**122**
	% Daily Value*
Total Fat 5.2g	7%
Saturated Fat 2.1g	10%
Cholesterol 15mg	5%
Sodium 460mg	20%
Total Carbohydrate 14g	5%
Dietary Fiber 3.3g	12%
Total Sugars 4g	
Protein 9.6g	
Vitamin D 0mcg	0%
Calcium 37mg	3%
Iron 1mg	7%
Potassium 433mg	9%

Russian Chicken Soup

A great, easy to cook Russian soup for cold winters. Great ingredients for IBD patients!

- Prep Time: 10 minutes
- Cook Time: 30 minutes
- Total Time: 40 minutes
- Serving: 6

Ingredients

- 3 lbs organic, grass-fed chicken breasts, cubed 1 inch (~2.54 cm)
- ¾ cup Capellini or gluten-free pasta
- 4 cups low-sodium chicken or vegetable broth, or water
- 1 tablespoon extra virgin olive oil
- 1 carrot, skin-removed and cubed 1 inch (~2.54 cm)
- 4 medium potatoes, cubed & peeled 1 inch (~2.54 cm)
- 2 tablespoons fresh lemon juice
- 1 bay leaf
- Salt and pepper, to taste

Instructions

1. Put all ingredients (except lemon juice and carrot) in a large pot and let it simmer over medium heat for 25 minutes.
2. Add carrots and lemon juice to the soup. Cook it for five more minutes. Then, adjust salt and pepper as desired.
3. Enjoy!

Cooking Tips:

- If you are in remission, you can fry chicken and carrot in a pan by one tablespoon of extra virgin olive oil and 1-teaspoon turmeric powder until golden brown. Then add chicken and carrot to the soup.

Low residue diet-related Tips:

- Do not use pepper if you are experiencing a flare-up.

Nutrition Facts
Servings: 6

Amount per serving
Calories 276

	% Daily Value*
Total Fat 5g	6%
Saturated Fat 1.1g	5%
Cholesterol 66mg	22%
Sodium 70mg	3%
Total Carbohydrate 32.4g	12%
Dietary Fiber 3.8g	13%
Total Sugars 2.2g	
Protein 24.6g	
Vitamin D 0mcg	0%
Calcium 35mg	3%
Iron 2mg	11%
Potassium 779mg	17%

BABA GHANOUSH

A great vegetarian middle-eastern appetizer! You can serve Baba Ghanoush, hot or cold.

- Prep Time: 25 minutes
- Cook Time: 40 minutes
- Total Time: 65 minutes
- Serving: 4-6

Ingredients

- 2 eggplants, skin removed
- ¼ cup tahini
- 1 teaspoon extra virgin olive oil
- ½ tablespoon freshly squeezed lemon juice
- ¼ teaspoon salt
- ¼ teaspoon cumin powder
- 1 tablespoon fresh parsley, chopped (optional)

Instructions

1. Place eggplants, cut thin lengthwise into a baking sheet with olive oil. Prick all surfaces with a fork. Broil all sides until it gets golden brown and smell smoky.
2. Turn off the broiler. Heat eggplants in the oven in a 375 °F. Let the eggplants roast for 30 minutes.
3. Remove eggplants from the oven. Cool down for 10 minutes and then add the tahini, lemon juice, cumin powder and salt to it.
4. Mash the roasted mix with a fork until getting a great smooth texture.
5. Drizzle a little bit of olive oil and fresh parsley on top. Enjoy!

Cooking Tips:

- You can use roasted zucchini instead of the eggplants as well.

Low residue diet-related Tips:

- Do not use pepper if you are experiencing a severe flare-up.
- It is better to use the eggplants with no seeds/fewer seeds, especially if you have complications such as large intestinal strictures.

```
Nutrition Facts
Servings: 4
Amount per serving
Calories                         168
                        % Daily Value*
Total Fat 9.8g                   13%
  Saturated Fat 1.3g              7%
Cholesterol 0mg                   0%
Sodium 170mg                      7%
Total Carbohydrate 19.4g          7%
  Dietary Fiber 11.1g            40%
  Total Sugars 6.3g
Protein 5.3g
Vitamin D 0mcg                    0%
Calcium 90mg                      7%
Iron 2mg                         11%
Potassium 693mg                  15%
```

S*ALMON* B*RUSCHETTA*

Experience great tastes of salmon, bread, and cheese!

- Prep Time: 10 minutes
- Cook Time: 30 minutes
- Total Time: 40 minutes
- Serving: 4

Ingredients

- ½ cup smoked salmon, thinly sliced
- 8 baguette slices or gluten-free bread/baguette
- ½ cup low-fat cream cheese or lactose-free cheese such as Swiss
- 1 tablespoon grated horseradish
- 1 tablespoon fresh lemon juice

- 1 tablespoon extra virgin olive oil
- 1 cup Persian cucumbers, peeled & chopped
- 1 teaspoon lemon zest

Instructions

1. Cut your baguette to have 1-inch (~2.54 cm) pieces. Then, toast your baguette pieces.
2. Mix cheese, horseradish, olive oil, lemon juice, and zest in a bowl. Grate cucumbers in it.
3. Spread your mix on toast slices and put smoked salmon on top. Enjoy!

Cooking Tips:

- You can use toasts instead of baguette to have a delicious cold sandwich.

Nutrition Facts
Servings: 4

Amount per serving	
Calories	**224**
	% Daily Value*
Total Fat 14.8g	19%
Saturated Fat 7.2g	36%
Cholesterol 36mg	12%
Sodium 388mg	17%
Total Carbohydrate 14.9g	5%
Dietary Fiber 0.8g	3%
Total Sugars 1.1g	
Protein 8.2g	
Vitamin D 0mcg	0%
Calcium 38mg	3%
Iron 1mg	8%
Potassium 110mg	2%

GUACAMOLE-LIKE APPETIZER

A modified guacamole recipe for IBD patients.

- Prep Time: 5 minutes
- Cook Time: 0 minutes
- Total Time: 5 minutes

- Serving: 4-6

Ingredients

- 6 avocados, peeled
- ½ tablespoon extra virgin olive oil
- ¼ cup chopped fresh cilantro
- 2 tablespoons fresh lime juice
- 1 teaspoon fresh lemon juice
- ½ teaspoon salt

Instructions

1- In a large bowl, mash avocados.
2- Add extra virgin olive oil and other ingredients into it.
3- Enjoy!

Cooking Tips:

- You can serve guacamole with tacos if you can tolerate it.
- If you can tolerate tomatoes and onions (in small amounts), cube, and add them into your guacamole.

Low residue diet-related Tips:

- Do not use fresh cilantro if you are experiencing a severe flare-up. Do not take taco chips, as well.

Nutrition Facts	
Servings: 6	
Amount per serving	
Calories	**422**
	% Daily Value*
Total Fat 40.4g	52%
Saturated Fat 8.4g	42%
Cholesterol 0mg	0%
Sodium 207mg	9%
Total Carbohydrate 18g	7%
Dietary Fiber 13.5g	48%
Total Sugars 1.2g	
Protein 3.9g	
Vitamin D 0mcg	0%
Calcium 26mg	2%
Iron 1mg	7%
Potassium 988mg	21%

Homemade Lebanese Hummus

A healthy and tasty middle-eastern appetizer. An excellent option for vegetarians and IBD patients in remission.

- Prep Time: 5 minutes
- Cook Time: 60 minutes
- Total Time: 65 minutes
- Serving: 4

<u>Ingredients</u>

- ¼ lb dried chickpeas (soaked in water for one night)
- 1½ tablespoons tahini
- 1 tablespoon lemon juice
- 2 tablespoons extra virgin olive oil, divided
- ¼ teaspoon cumin
- ½ teaspoon salt
- 1 tablespoon water
- 1 teaspoon baking soda (optional)
- 1 teaspoon paprika powder (optional)

<u>Instructions</u>

1- First, IBD patients need to soak the chickpeas overnight in water and optionally add baking soda to the water.
2- Cook your chickpeas in a large pot with water over medium heat for about 1 hour. Check if chickpeas cooked well by crushing one of them with a fork in your hand.
3- When chickpeas cooked, drain them and put them in a blender.
4- Add 1 tablespoon of extra virgin olive oil, lemon juice, tahini, cumin powder and salt to the blender. Blend until your hummus gets a soft, creamy texture equally.
5- Sprinkle with 1 tablespoon extra virgin olive oil or paprika powder (optional).
6- Serve immediately or fridge it.

Cooking Tips:

- Hummus is well-matched with white pita bread.
- You can serve hummus, hot or cold.

Low residue diet-related Tips:

- Do not use paprika in hummus if you are experiencing a severe flare-up.
- Eat hummus in moderation when you are in remission. During a flare-up, it is better not to make this recipe or make and consume in a small amount.

Nutrition Facts	
Servings: 4	
Amount per serving	
Calories	**198**
	% Daily Value*
Total Fat 11.8g	15%
Saturated Fat 1.6g	8%
Cholesterol 0mg	0%
Sodium 305mg	13%
Total Carbohydrate 18.5g	7%
Dietary Fiber 5.5g	20%
Total Sugars 3.1g	
Protein 6.5g	
Vitamin D 0mcg	0%
Calcium 56mg	4%
Iron 2mg	13%
Potassium 279mg	6%

Crab Dip with Wonton Chips

A great, easy-to-make appetizer with crabs in wonton wrappers!

- Prep Time: 5 minutes
- Cook Time: 30 minutes
- Total Time: 35 minutes
- Serving: 6

Ingredients

- 1 package Wonton wrappers or gluten-free wonton wrappers
- 1 teaspoon extra virgin olive oil
- 1 can crab meat, chopped
- ½ cup organic mayonnaise
- 1 tablespoon soy sauce
- ½ cup cream cheese or lactose-free cheese
- ½ teaspoon lemon juice
- 1 scallion, chopped
- 1 tablespoon honey or maple syrup
- 1 teaspoon salt, divided
- ½ teaspoon black pepper (optional)

Instructions

1- Preheat oven to 400 °F.
2- Mix all ingredients into a large mixing bowl. Stir well.
3- In a baking dish, pour all the mix and bake for 30 minutes until you see edge bubbles.
4- Diagonally cut wonton wrappers in half and make triangles. Alternatively, you can make wonton cups.
5- Pour the cups with your mix.
6- Spray extra virgin olive oil on a baking sheet. Put triangles on it and spray olive oil on wontons as well. Add salt as desired. Let the wontons bake for 7 minutes until golden brown.
7- Remove from the oven. Serve and Enjoy!

Cooking Tips:

- You need to watch wontons while baking carefully. They can be burnt fast.
- You can have one teaspoon of stevia instead of honey or maple syrup if you cannot tolerate them.

Low residue diet-related Tips:

- Do not use pepper if you are experiencing a severe flare-up.
- When during a flare-up, boil scallion first and then add it to the mix.

Nutrition Facts	
Servings: 6	
Amount per serving	
Calories	**223**
	% Daily Value*
Total Fat 14.5g	19%
Saturated Fat 5.4g	27%
Cholesterol 46mg	15%
Sodium 881mg	38%
Total Carbohydrate 16.2g	6%
Dietary Fiber 0.3g	1%
Total Sugars 4.3g	
Protein 7.5g	
Vitamin D 0mcg	0%
Calcium 48mg	4%
Iron 1mg	6%
Potassium 129mg	3%

SHRIMP SALAD

Are you looking for a delicious salad with shrimp? You can follow this recipe to have one!

- Prep Time: 5 minutes
- Cook Time: 15 minutes
- Total Time: 20 minutes
- Serving: 2-4

Ingredients

- 1 lb shrimp, peeled
- 1 celery stalk, chopped
- 1 tablespoon extra virgin olive oil
- 1 tablespoon fresh lemon juice
- ½ teaspoon turmeric powder
- Salt and pepper, to taste
- 2 tablespoons organic low-fat mayonnaise (optional)

Instructions

1. Cook shrimps by extra virgin olive oil and turmeric in a medium pan over medium heat.

2. In a large bowl, mix all lemon juice, salt, pepper, and mayonnaise (optional).
3. Add cooked shrimp to the bowl and combine.
4. Serve and enjoy!

Cooking Tips:

- You can prepare your shrimps in the oven as well. Just preheat oven to 375 °F. Choose a cooking sheet and spray olive oil on it. Put shrimp on your cooking sheet and let it cook until golden brown (around 10 minutes).

Low residue diet-related Tips:

- Do not use pepper and mayonnaise if you are experiencing a flare-up.

Nutrition Facts
Servings: 4

Amount per serving	
Calories	**197**
	% Daily Value*
Total Fat 8g	10%
Saturated Fat 1.5g	7%
Cholesterol 241mg	80%
Sodium 347mg	15%
Total Carbohydrate 3.9g	1%
Dietary Fiber 0.2g	1%
Total Sugars 0.6g	
Protein 26g	
Vitamin D 0mcg	0%
Calcium 107mg	8%
Iron 1mg	3%
Potassium 217mg	5%

Zucchini Salad (Spiralized)

A great summer salad based on a zucchini. Zucchini salad is a healthy choice for IBD patients.

- Prep Time: 30 minutes
- Total Time: 30 minutes

- Serving: 2-4

Ingredients

- 2 zucchinis, chopped
- ¼ cup low-fat/fat-free feta cheese or lactose-free aged cheddar
- 1 tablespoon extra virgin olive oil
- 2 tablespoons fresh lemon juice
- 1 tablespoon parsley, chopped (optional)
- Salt and pepper, to taste

Instructions

1. Make spiral zucchinis or cut them thin and lengthwise
2. In a large bowl, mix zucchinis and all other ingredients.
3. For better taste, let it rest for 15 minutes. Enjoy!

Cooking Tips:

- You can use vegetable peelers if you do not have a spiralizer.

Low residue diet-related Tips:

- Do not use pepper if you are experiencing a severe flare-up.
- Check if you can tolerate fresh parsley well or not. If you cannot tolerate, remove it from the recipe.

Nutrition Facts

Servings: 4

Amount per serving

Calories 65

	% Daily Value*
Total Fat 3.7g	5%
Saturated Fat 0.6g	3%
Cholesterol 2mg	1%
Sodium 141mg	6%
Total Carbohydrate 3.9g	1%
Dietary Fiber 1.1g	4%
Total Sugars 1.9g	
Protein 4.8g	
Vitamin D 0mcg	0%
Calcium 65mg	5%
Iron 0mg	2%
Potassium 266mg	6%

OLIVIER SALAD (CHICKEN, POTATO & EGG SALAD)

A traditional well-known Russian salad with great ingredients for IBD patients. For having a better taste, you can refrigerate it for 30 minutes.

- Prep Time: 15 minutes
- Cook Time: 45 minutes
- Total Time: 60 minutes
- Serving: 6

Ingredients

- 4 potatoes, skin removed and chopped
- 2 cups chicken breasts, shredded
- 2 organic, free-range eggs
- 2 medium carrots
- 2 tablespoons extra virgin olive oil
- 2 tablespoons fresh lemon juice
- 1 cup organic low-fat mayonnaise
- Salt and pepper, to taste

Instructions

1. Cook eggs, potatoes, and carrots in a large pot over medium/high heat. Use enough water to cover all ingredients.
2. Mash potatoes and eggs. Cube carrots (0.3-inch size).
3. In a large bowl, mix all ingredients well.
4. Refrigerate it for 10-15 minutes. Enjoy!

Cooking Tips:

- You can cube your potatoes and eggs similar to carrots, instead of mashing them.

Low residue diet-related Tips:

- Do not use pepper and mayonnaise if you are experiencing a flare-up.
- Always use mayo in moderation. If you cannot tolerate, use plain yogurt or lactose-free plain yogurt.

Nutrition Facts

Servings: 6

Amount per serving

Calories	300
	% Daily Value*
Total Fat 10.2g	13%
Saturated Fat 2.2g	11%
Cholesterol 111mg	37%
Sodium 931mg	40%
Total Carbohydrate 28.6g	10%
Dietary Fiber 4.4g	16%
Total Sugars 5.5g	
Protein 23.8g	
Vitamin D 5mcg	26%
Calcium 40mg	3%
Iron 2mg	11%
Potassium 758mg	16%

Apple-Pear Salad with A Special Vinaigrette

A simple great fruit salad for everyone!

- Prep Time: 10 minutes
- Total Time: 10 minutes

- Serving: 4-6

Ingredients

- 3 cooked pears, peeled and chopped
- 1 papaya, peeled and chopped
- 3 apples, peeled and chopped
- ¼ cup honey or maple syrup
- 3 tablespoons fresh lemon juice
- ¼ cup fresh mint leaves, chopped (optional)

Instructions

1. Add all your ingredients in a large bowl and mix well.
2. Serve cold. Enjoy!

Cooking Tips:

- Remove honey or maple syrup from ingredients if you cannot tolerate any of them.

Low residue diet-related Tips:

- Check if you can tolerate fresh mint leaves or not. Remove from ingredients if you cannot tolerate it.

Nutrition Facts

Servings: 4

Amount per serving

Calories 278

	% Daily Value*
Total Fat 0.8g	1%
Saturated Fat 0.1g	1%
Cholesterol 0mg	0%
Sodium 13mg	1%
Total Carbohydrate 73.2g	27%
Dietary Fiber 10.4g	37%
Total Sugars 56.5g	
Protein 1.6g	
Vitamin D 0mcg	0%
Calcium 33mg	3%
Iron 1mg	7%
Potassium 529mg	11%

Beet, Carrot & Apple Salad

A colorful salad with amazing fruits and vegetables inside!

- Prep Time: 10 minutes
- Total Time: 10 minutes
- Serving: 4-6

Ingredients

- 1 lb beet, peeled and cubed 1 inch (~2.54 cm)
- 2 medium carrots, peeled and cubed 1 inch (~2.54 cm)
- 1 apple, peeled and cubed 1 inch (~2.54 cm)
- 3 tablespoons fresh orange juice
- 2 tablespoons fresh lime juice
- 1 tablespoon extra virgin olive oil
- Salt and pepper, to taste
- ¼ cup fresh mint leaves, chopped (optional)

Instructions

1. In a large bowl, mix well all ingredients.
2. Serve cold. Enjoy!

Cooking Tips:

- Wear gloves to cover your hands when you cut beets.

Low residue diet-related Tips:

- Check if you can tolerate fresh mint leaves or not. Remove from ingredients if you cannot tolerate it.
- Do not use pepper if you are experiencing a severe flare-up.

- Cook beets or remove it from ingredients when you are experiencing a flare-up.

Nutrition Facts	
Servings: 4	
Amount per serving	
Calories	**129**
	% Daily Value*
Total Fat 3.8g	5%
Saturated Fat 0.5g	3%
Cholesterol 0mg	0%
Sodium 109mg	5%
Total Carbohydrate 24.1g	9%
Dietary Fiber 4.4g	16%
Total Sugars 17.5g	
Protein 2.4g	
Vitamin D 0mcg	0%
Calcium 30mg	2%
Iron 1mg	8%
Potassium 539mg	11%

Butter Lettuce Salad with Honey Vinaigrette

A light and delicious salad for IBD patients who can tolerate butter lettuce with a delicious dressing.

- Prep Time: 15 minutes
- Total Time: 15 minutes
- Serving: 4-6

Ingredients

- 2 medium butter lettuces, cut into small pieces (also called Bibb, Boston or living lettuce)
- 1 tablespoon honey or maple syrup
- 2 tablespoons fresh lemon juice
- 2 tablespoons fresh lime juice
- 2 tablespoons extra virgin olive oil
- Salt and pepper to taste

Instructions

1. Wash butter lettuce thoroughly and cut into small pieces
2. In a large bowl, mix well all ingredients.
3. Serve cold. Enjoy!

Cooking Tips:

- You can add two peeled Persian cucumbers to have a garden-like salad!

Low residue diet-related Tips:

- Butter lettuce, also called Bibb, living or Boston lettuce, is a type of lettuce that can be digested easier than other types of lettuce. Hence, it is an excellent option for IBD patients to try butter lettuce and check if they can tolerate it or not. Many of IBD patients can enjoy a garden salad with butter lettuce during remissions.
- Do not use pepper if you are experiencing a severe flare-up.

Nutrition Facts
Servings: 4

Amount per serving
Calories 91

	% Daily Value*
Total Fat 7.1g	9%
Saturated Fat 1.1g	5%
Cholesterol 0mg	0%
Sodium 21mg	1%
Total Carbohydrate 7.5g	3%
Dietary Fiber 1.1g	4%
Total Sugars 5.7g	
Protein 1.2g	
Vitamin D 0mcg	0%
Calcium 33mg	3%
Iron 0mg	1%
Potassium 237mg	5%

CARROT-AVOCADO SALAD

An epic salad recipe with avocado and tasty dressing. A great salad option for IBD patients!

- Prep Time: 20 minutes
- Cook Time: 30 minutes
- Total Time: 50 minutes
- Serving: 4-6

Ingredients

- 1 large avocado
- 2 carrots, peeled and diced 1-inch (~2.54 cm)
- 2 tablespoons extra virgin olive oil
- 1 tablespoon fresh lemon juice
- Salt and pepper, to taste
- ⅓ cup green onion, chopped (optional)
- ¼ cup fresh mint leaves, chopped (optional)

Instructions

1. Peel-off carrots.
2. In a small pot, cook carrots in boiling water over medium heat.
3. Cube carrots and avocados. In a medium bowl, mix other ingredients and then add carrot and avocado.
4. Mix well. Enjoy!

Cooking Tips:

- You can cook carrots in a small pan with one tablespoon of extra virgin olive oil and ½ teaspoon of turmeric powder over medium heat as well.

Low residue diet-related Tips:

- Make sure your gut can tolerate green onion before using it.
- Do not use pepper, green onion, and fresh mint if you are experiencing a flare-up.

Nutrition Facts
Servings: 4

Amount per serving	
Calories	**179**
	% Daily Value*
Total Fat 16.9g	22%
Saturated Fat 3.1g	15%
Cholesterol 0mg	0%
Sodium 26mg	1%
Total Carbohydrate 8g	3%
Dietary Fiber 4.4g	16%
Total Sugars 2g	
Protein 1.4g	
Vitamin D 0mcg	0%
Calcium 22mg	2%
Iron 1mg	3%
Potassium 369mg	8%

Classic Tuna Pasta Salad

Classic tuna with pasta is an excellent choice as your salad. You can have it for lunch or dinner as well.

- Prep Time: 15 minutes
- Cook Time: 15 minutes
- Total Time: 30 minutes
- Serving: 4

Ingredients

- 1½ cups pasta (rotini preferred), or gluten-free pasta
- 1 celery stalk, chopped
- 1 can tuna in water
- ½ cup organic low-fat mayonnaise
- 2 tablespoons lemon juice
- Salt and pepper, to taste

Instructions

1. Cook pasta according to its package instruction.
2. Drain pasta and place it in a large bowl.
3. Add celery, tuna, and all other ingredients to the pasta bowl. Mix well.
4. It is better to let it cool in the fridge for 30 minutes. Enjoy!

<u>Low residue diet-related Tips:</u>

- Do not use pepper if you are experiencing a flare-up.

Nutrition Facts	
Servings: 4	
Amount per serving	
Calories	**105**
	% Daily Value*
Total Fat 3g	4%
Saturated Fat 0.7g	3%
Cholesterol 25mg	8%
Sodium 526mg	23%
Total Carbohydrate 8.9g	3%
Dietary Fiber 1.4g	5%
Total Sugars 4.9g	
Protein 10.4g	
Vitamin D 0mcg	0%
Calcium 13mg	1%
Iron 1mg	3%
Potassium 159mg	3%

SALMON CEVICHE

This salad is full of omega-3 with a fabulous dressing. Enjoy this dairy-free, egg-free, nut-free, and gluten-free recipe.

- Prep Time: 15 minutes
- Rest Time: 15 minutes
- Total Time: 30 minutes
- Serving: 4

<u>Ingredients</u>

- 1 lb salmon, skin removed and cubed

- 1 cup Persian cucumber, cubed 1cm
- ½ cup green onion, chopped well
- 1 tablespoon fresh lemon juice
- 1 tablespoon fresh lime juice
- 1 tablespoon grated fresh ginger
- Salt and pepper, to taste
- 1 teaspoon dried oregano (optional)

Instructions

1. In a large bowl, mix salmon, cucumber, green onion, ginger, and oregano.
2. In a small cup/bowl, whisk lime & lemon juice, salt, and pepper and pour it into the large bowl.
3. Mix all well. Serve cold. Enjoy!

Cooking Tips:

- You can add ½ teaspoon freshly grated turmeric if you want to enjoy its anti-inflammatory properties.

Low residue diet-related Tips:

- Make sure your gut can tolerate green onion and oregano before using them.
- Do not use pepper if you are experiencing a flare-up.

Nutrition Facts	
Servings: 4	
Amount per serving	
Calories	**167**
	% Daily Value*
Total Fat 7.1g	9%
Saturated Fat 1.1g	5%
Cholesterol 50mg	17%
Sodium 53mg	2%
Total Carbohydrate 3.9g	1%
Dietary Fiber 1.1g	4%
Total Sugars 0.8g	
Protein 22.4g	
Vitamin D 0mcg	0%
Calcium 52mg	4%
Iron 1mg	6%
Potassium 506mg	11%

HONEY CHICKEN SALAD

Enjoy making a rich salad with chicken and honey. Excellent source of protein for IBD patients.

- Prep Time: 25 minutes
- Total Time: 25 minutes
- Serving: 4-6

Ingredients

- 1 lb chicken breasts, skinless and boneless
- 1 avocado, chopped
- 4 tablespoons honey or maple syrup
- 6 cups butter lettuce, chopped
- 3 tablespoons lemon juice
- 1 tablespoon low-fat feta cheese or lactose-free aged cheddar
- 2 tablespoons extra virgin olive oil
- Salt and pepper, to taste
- 1 tablespoon green onion, chopped (optional)

Instructions

1. In a large pan, cook chickens with two tablespoons of extra virgin olive oil over medium heat until getting close to a golden brown. Remove from pan and cut into 1-inch (~2.54 cm) cubes.
2. In a large bowl, whisk honey (or maple syrup), lemon juice, green onion (optional), cheese, salt, and pepper.
3. In another large bowl, cut lettuce into small pieces. Add cubed chickens and pour the sauce on top. Serve and enjoy!

Cooking Tips:

- You can boil chickens in a pot over medium heat (recommended for flare-up times).
- If you cannot tolerate honey, use maple syrup or agave syrup instead.

Low residue diet-related Tips:

- Make sure your gut can tolerate green onion before using it.
- Do not use pepper if you are experiencing a flare-up.

Nutrition Facts
Servings: 6

Amount per serving	
Calories	**310**
	% Daily Value*
Total Fat 17.1g	22%
Saturated Fat 3.6g	18%
Cholesterol 68mg	23%
Sodium 152mg	7%
Total Carbohydrate 16.5g	6%
Dietary Fiber 2.8g	10%
Total Sugars 12.3g	
Protein 23.6g	
Vitamin D 0mcg	0%
Calcium 29mg	2%
Iron 3mg	15%
Potassium 444mg	9%

Main Courses

Mediterranean Chicken - Zucchini Stew

Chicken–Zucchini stew is one of the delicious Mediterranean stews, which typically serves with steamed white rice. Turmeric, zucchini, and white rice are great for IBD patients, and most can well-tolerate them.

- Prep Time: 10 minutes
- Cook Time: 50 minutes
- Total Time: 60 minutes
- Serving: 4

Ingredients

- 4 Fresh zucchinis, lengthwise-cut with no skin
- 6 Skin-removed chicken legs
- 4 tablespoons extra virgin olive oil
- 1.5 teaspoon turmeric
- ½ teaspoon black pepper
- 1½ teaspoons salt
- 3 tablespoons lemon juice or 1 lime
- 2½ cups water
- 4 tablespoons tomato paste (optional)

Preparation

1. Fry, both sides of skinless zucchinis with two tablespoons of extra virgin olive oil in a sauté pan until golden brown.
2. In another pan, fry your chicken legs with the rest of extra virgin olive oil, salt, pepper, and turmeric until golden brown.

3. Boil water in a pot and dissolve tomato paste to the boiling water if you want (optional). Stir well.
4. Add your chicken legs to the boiling water. Turn the heat to medium. Let it simmer for 20 minutes. If your sauce gets thick, add more water to your stew.
5. After 25 minutes, add your zucchinis and your lemon juice to the stew and let it cook for another 5 minutes. After three minutes, taste your stew and correct your seasonings. Do not add more black peppers.
6. Enjoy this meal with steamed white rice!

Cooking Tips:

- To reach a faster cooking time, you can add all the ingredients into the boiling water and let the stew cook for 40 minutes on high heat.
- You can use eggplant instead of zucchini to make a delicious Eggplant Stew. Just remember not to use the eggplants seeds or remove eggplant small edible seeds.

Low residue diet-related Tips:

- Some IBD patients cannot tolerate tomato pastes. In that case, cook this stew without tomato paste or use two cups of organic beef bone broth instead of water.
- If you are in a flare-up, try not to use pepper and remove zucchini's skins.
- If you have a colon stricture, try not to alternate zucchini with eggplant with lots of seeds.

Nutrition Facts
Servings: 4

Amount per serving	
Calories	**352**
	% Daily Value*
Total Fat 22.6g	29%
Saturated Fat 4.4g	22%
Cholesterol 89mg	30%
Sodium 1001mg	44%
Total Carbohydrate 10.5g	4%
Dietary Fiber 3.1g	11%
Total Sugars 5.6g	
Protein 28.9g	
Vitamin D 0mcg	0%
Calcium 55mg	4%
Iron 3mg	16%
Potassium 945mg	20%

LACTOSE-FREE CHICKEN FETTUCCINE ALFREDO

Do you love to have a creamy-but-healthy Fettuccine Alfredo? You can use this recipe to have a delicious Italian main course. This meal has chicken/vegetable stock, turmeric, ginger, and lemon that are great for IBD patients.

- Prep Time: 15 minutes
- Cook Time: 30 minutes
- Total Time: 45 minutes
- Serving: 4

Ingredients

- 4 boneless, skinless chicken breasts, about 0.8 inches (~2 cm) thick
- ¾ lb uncooked fettuccine (~340 g) or gluten-free fettuccine/pasta
- 3 tablespoons all-purpose flour or gluten-free flour
- 10 oz lactose-free milk (~300 ml)
- ½ cup unsalted organic chicken stock or vegetable stock (~120 ml)
- 1 tablespoon fresh lemon juice
- 3½ teaspoons Himalayan salt, divided

- 2 teaspoons black pepper, divided
- 1 teaspoon turmeric
- 1 teaspoon ginger powder
- 3 tablespoons extra virgin olive oil, divided
- Fresh parsley, minced (optional)

Preparation

1. Heat a tablespoon of extra virgin olive oil in a pan. Add your chicken breast with one tablespoon of salt, one tablespoon of pepper and turmeric and let it cook for 5 minutes until golden brown both sides.
2. Boil the water in a large pot over high heat. Add one tablespoon of high-quality extra virgin olive oil and one tablespoon of salt to the water. Then, add your fettuccine in the boiling water.
3. Cook fettuccine according to its package instructions. Drain and return to the pot.
4. In another pan, put one tablespoon of extra virgin olive oil on medium heat. When heated, add your flour slowly and whisk until golden brown.
5. Heat your lactose-free milk in the microwave, add it slowly to your flour, and whisk for 3 minutes. Add lemon juice, ginger powder, one tablespoon of pepper, and one tablespoon of salt to make an excellent béchamel sauce.
6. Add chicken/vegetable stock to the béchamel sauce, frequently stir for 10 minutes until thickened.
7. Slice or cube chicken. Add the béchamel sauce to your fettuccine pot and toss perfectly.
8. Garnish the top with minced parsley and enjoy!

Cooking Tips:

- If you are not lactose-intolerant, you can use regular cow milk.
- If you are gluten intolerant, you can use gluten-free pasta/fettuccine.

Low residue diet-related Tips:

- Do not use parsley if you cannot tolerate it.
- Make sure that your chickens are skinless.
- If you are in a flare-up, try not to use pepper.

Nutrition Facts	
Servings: 4	
Amount per serving	
Calories	**626**
	% Daily Value*
Total Fat 23.2g	30%
Saturated Fat 5.1g	25%
Cholesterol 170mg	57%
Sodium 2433mg	106%
Total Carbohydrate 51g	19%
Dietary Fiber 3.6g	13%
Total Sugars 1.3g	
Protein 50.5g	
Vitamin D 0mcg	0%
Calcium 52mg	4%
Iron 4mg	20%
Potassium 387mg	8%

Chicken with Mashed Potatoes

For those who want a very simple but delicious main course. Cooked baby carrot can be used as a well-matched garnish.

- Prep Time: 5 minutes
- Cook Time: 20 minutes
- Total Time: 25 minutes
- Serving: 4

Ingredients

- 4 skinless, boneless chicken breast

- 2 tablespoons extra virgin olive oil, divided
- 1½ cups unsalted chicken stock (organic preferred)
- 2 skin-removed large potatoes
- ½ cup lactose-free milk
- 1 teaspoon black pepper, divided
- ¼ teaspoon salt, divided
- ¼ teaspoon turmeric
- 1 tablespoon minced parsley (optional)

<u>Preparation</u>

1. High-heat 2 tablespoons of extra virgin olive oil in a pan. Add your chicken breast with ½ tablespoon of salt, pepper, and one tablespoon of turmeric and let it cook until golden brown both sides.
2. Cook all potatoes in a medium pot with a little pinch of turmeric.
3. Mash your potatoes and add the rest of salt and pepper.
4. Heat lactose-free milk in the microwave and add to your mashed potato. Whisk well.
5. Pour your plate with mashed potato, and chicken on top.

<u>Cooking Tips:</u>

- If you are not lactose-intolerant, you can use low-fat normal cow whole milk.
- You can make the Béchamel sauce (explained before in Fettuccine Alfredo recipe) and add it to your chicken and mashed potato.

<u>Low residue diet-related Tips:</u>

- Do not use parsley if you cannot tolerate it.

- Make sure that your chickens and potatoes are skinless as IBD patients may not tolerate skins
- If you are in a flare-up, try not to use pepper.

Nutrition Facts

Servings: 4

Amount per serving

Calories   **448**

	% Daily Value*
Total Fat 15.8g	20%
Saturated Fat 3.1g	16%
Cholesterol 108mg	36%
Sodium 279mg	12%
Total Carbohydrate 33g	12%
Dietary Fiber 3.3g	12%
Total Sugars 3.1g	
Protein 42.8g	
Vitamin D 0mcg	0%
Calcium 49mg	4%
Iron 3mg	14%
Potassium 911mg	19%

CHICKEN STROGANOFF

Try Chicken Stroganoff with potatoes and incredible gravy, matched with patient's tolerance levels.

- Prep Time: 5 minutes
- Cook Time: 15 minutes
- Total Time: 20 minutes
- Serving: 4

<u>Ingredients</u>

- 4 skinless, boneless chicken breast
- 2 tablespoons all-purpose flour or gluten-free flour
- 2 cups (~500 ml) unsalted/salt-reduced beef broth (organic preferred)
- 1 tablespoon of salt and pepper
- 3 tablespoons extra virgin olive oil
- ⅓ cup lactose-free milk
- 1 tablespoon fresh lemon juice

- ½ tablespoon ginger powder or fresh ginger
- ½ tablespoon turmeric
- 10 oz (~300 gr) mushrooms, thickly sliced
- Parsley, minced (optional)

Instructions

1. Heat a tablespoon of high-quality extra virgin olive oil in a pan. Flat your chicken breasts and cook them with ½ tablespoon of salt, ½ tablespoon of pepper and ginger powder until golden brown both sides.
2. In another pan, put one tablespoon of extra virgin olive oil on medium heat. When heated, sauté your mushrooms. Then, add your flour slowly and whisk until golden brown.
3. Heat your lactose-free milk in the microwave, add it slowly to your flour, and whisk for 3 minutes. Add lemon juice, ½ tablespoon of pepper, and ½ tablespoon of salt to make a great sauce. Stir the sauce on low heat until it becomes thick.
4. Fry very thin-sliced potatoes with one tablespoon of extra virgin olive oil and ½ tablespoon of turmeric.
5. Add your fries and chicken to your sauce. Let it cook for two more minutes.
6. Garnish the top with minced parsley and enjoy!

Cooking Tips:

- If you are not lactose-intolerant, you can use low-fat cow whole milk.
- You can use pork tenderloin or turkey breast instead of chicken breast.
- If you like, you can serve it with any pasta as well.

Low residue diet-related Tips:

- Make sure that your chickens and potatoes are skinless as IBD patients may not tolerate skins.
- If you are in a flare-up, try not to use pepper.
- If you are in a flare-up, try to Airfry your fries or boil them.
- Do not use mushrooms or parsley if you cannot tolerate them.

Nutrition Facts	
Servings: 4	
Amount per serving	
Calories	**274**
	% Daily Value*
Total Fat 13.2g	17%
Saturated Fat 1.9g	10%
Cholesterol 67mg	22%
Sodium 433mg	19%
Total Carbohydrate 10.7g	4%
Dietary Fiber 2.6g	9%
Total Sugars 2.7g	
Protein 29.8g	
Vitamin D 15mcg	77%
Calcium 42mg	3%
Iron 3mg	17%
Potassium 331mg	7%

Chicken Kebab

Enjoy a classic barbecued chicken, well-marinated in saffron and yogurt!

- Prep Time: 15 minutes
- (Marinate Time: 2 hours)
- Cook Time: 25 minutes
- Total Time: 40 minutes
- Serving: 4

Ingredients

- 4 chicken breasts, cut into 1.5 inches (3.8) cubes
- ¾ cup lactose-free yogurt or plain yogurt if you are not lactose intolerant
- 1 large onion

- ¼ cup saffron (bloomed)
- 1 tablespoon salt
- 3 tablespoons extra virgin olive oil
- 1 tablespoon lemon juice

Instructions

1. Cut your onions and make onion rings.
2. To marinate your chicken, mix and stir it well with onion, lactose-free plain yogurt, bloomed saffron, olive oil, salt, and lemon juice together (To have a bloomed saffron, you need to grind your saffron perfectly and add 100ml of boiling water to it).
3. Cover the marinated bowl and put it in the fridge to rest for two hours.
4. After two hours, thread chickens into skewers and grilled both sides well until golden brown

Cooking Tips:

- If you are not lactose-intolerant, you can use low-fat plain yogurt.
- You can use the oven instead of grilling chickens. Just preheat the oven to 400 °F, cover chickens with aluminum foils, and let it cook for about 25 minutes. Use broil for five minutes if you want a golden brown texture.
- You can use chicken with bones instead of chicken breasts, as well.

Low residue diet-related Tips:

- If you cannot tolerate saffron (rarely happens), do not add saffron to chicken. Instead, put ⅓ tablespoon of turmeric.

Nutrition Facts
Servings: 4

Amount per serving	
Calories	**322**
	% Daily Value*
Total Fat 21g	27%
Saturated Fat 2.5g	12%
Cholesterol 68mg	23%
Sodium 1812mg	79%
Total Carbohydrate 7.4g	3%
Dietary Fiber 0.9g	3%
Total Sugars 1.7g	
Protein 27.6g	
Vitamin D 0mcg	0%
Calcium 70mg	5%
Iron 0mg	2%
Potassium 174mg	4%

ROASTED CHICKEN WITH POMEGRANATE SAUCE

Have you tried a sour taste of chicken with pomegranate sauce? This dish is an excellent sample of a delicious sour chicken. You can make your dish sweet and sour by adding honey to the recipe.

- Prep Time: 10 minutes
- (Marinate Time: 2 hours)
- Cook Time: 40 minutes
- Total Time: 50 minutes
- Serving: 4

Ingredients

- 4 Chicken legs and thighs, skinless
- ¼ cup bloomed saffron
- 2 tablespoons extra virgin olive oil
- 5 tablespoons lime juice
- ½ cup pomegranate sauce
- 1 tablespoon salt
- 1 tablespoon turmeric
- 2 cups of water
- ½ tablespoon Black pepper

- ½ cup honey (optional)

Instructions

1. In a large bowl, marinate your chicken with bloomed saffron, lime juice, honey (optional) salt and pepper.
2. Mix and stir all ingredients well. Cover the bowl top and fridge it for 2 hours.
3. Roast your chicken with extra virgin olive oil and turmeric for 15 minutes until golden brown.
4. Boil two cups of water and add pomegranate sauce. Stir well until dissolved.
5. Put your chicken in the sauce and let it cook for 25 minutes. Let the sauce thicken, and then you are done!
6. Serve it with white basmati rice and enjoy!

Cooking Tips:

- Alternatively, you may want to use chicken breasts instead of chicken legs and thighs.
- If you do not find the pomegranate sauce or paste, you can add 200ml of pomegranate juice. It makes your meal hard to be thickened, but it gives you a similar taste.

Low residue diet-related Tips:

- If you cannot tolerate saffron (rarely happens), do not add saffron to chicken. Instead, put ⅓ tablespoon of turmeric.
- Pomegranate has anti-inflammatory properties, which is excellent for IBD patients, and it can be well-tolerate in many patients. However, if you cannot

tolerate it, use dark grape juice instead. Make sure pomegranates are consumed seedless.

Nutrition Facts	
Servings: 4	
Amount per serving	
Calories	**303**
	% Daily Value*
Total Fat 17.2g	22%
Saturated Fat 3.6g	18%
Cholesterol 90mg	30%
Sodium 2094mg	91%
Total Carbohydrate 16.4g	6%
Dietary Fiber 0.6g	2%
Total Sugars 11.4g	
Protein 22.7g	
Vitamin D 0mcg	0%
Calcium 33mg	3%
Iron 2mg	13%
Potassium 79mg	2%

Puffy Chicken

A tremendous yummy puffy chicken strips for adults and kids.

- Prep Time: 10 minutes
- Cook Time: 20 minutes
- Total Time: 30 minutes
- Serving: 4

<u>Ingredients</u>

- 4 strip cuts of chicken breast (~400 grams)
- 150 grams of all-purpose flour or gluten-free flour
- 5 tablespoons alcohol-free carbonated malt drink
- 2 tablespoons extra virgin olive oil
- 3 eggs (organic range-free preferred)
- ½ tablespoon salt
- ½ tablespoon turmeric powder
- ½ teaspoon stevia or maple syrup (optional)
- 1 tablespoon active dried yeast (optional)

Instructions

1. In a large bowl, marinate your chicken with malt drink, yeast, olive oil, salt, and turmeric. Mix all well.
2. In another bowl, whisk all three eggs perfectly.
3. First, deep your marinated chickens into eggs and then cover it with flour.
4. Cook your chicken in a pan over medium heat with extra virgin olive oil.

Cooking Tips:

- You can use stevia or maple syrup to give a sweet taste to your dish.
- Instead of carbonated malt drink, you can use carbonated water. In this case, you need to use active dry yeast.

Low residue diet-related Tips:

- If you are in a flare-up, put your marinated chicken in boiling water instead of frying it.
- If you can tolerate beer a little bit, you can use it instead of malt drink.
- This dish is well-matched with Tartar sauce. So, if you tolerate Tartar, enjoy this meal with it!

Nutrition Facts	
Servings: 4	
Amount per serving	
Calories	**458**
	% Daily Value*
Total Fat 16g	20%
Saturated Fat 3.5g	18%
Cholesterol 221mg	74%
Sodium 1051mg	46%
Total Carbohydrate 31.8g	12%
Dietary Fiber 1.3g	5%
Total Sugars 2g	
Protein 44.3g	
Vitamin D 12mcg	58%
Calcium 46mg	4%
Iron 4mg	22%
Potassium 410mg	9%

CHICKEN SCALOPPINI

Enjoy a delicious Italian dish with ingredients great for IBD patients!

- Prep Time: 10 minutes
- Cook Time: 15 minutes
- Total Time: 25 minutes
- Serving: 4

Ingredients

- 4 skinless and boneless chicken breast
- 2 teaspoons fresh lemon juice
- 1 tablespoon extra virgin olive oil
- 6 tablespoons bread crumbs or any gluten-free dried bread
- ½ cup unsalted, no-fat chicken broth
- 1 tablespoon lime juice
- 1 tablespoon well-cooked capers
- ¼ teaspoon salt
- ¼ teaspoon black pepper

Instructions

1. First, use a meat mallet to pound your chicken breasts.
2. Add lemon juice, salt, and pepper to your chicken
3. Heat a pan with extra virgin olive oil over medium heat. Add your chicken to the pan and cook each side for about 5 minutes until golden brown.
4. In the end, add chicken broth and your breadcrumbs and stir well for five more minutes until it gets thick.
5. Garnish with capers. Enjoy!

Low residue diet-related Tips:

- Make sure you cooked capers well.
- Just use peppers if you can tolerate them.
- If you are in a flare-up, do not need to fry chicken. Just boil it in chicken broth.

Nutrition Facts
Servings: 4

Amount per serving
Calories: 320

	% Daily Value*
Total Fat 11g	14%
Saturated Fat 2.6g	13%
Cholesterol 35mg	12%
Sodium 863mg	38%
Total Carbohydrate 33.2g	12%
Dietary Fiber 1.5g	6%
Total Sugars 0.7g	
Protein 20.6g	
Vitamin D 0mcg	0%
Calcium 19mg	1%
Iron 2mg	9%
Potassium 28mg	1%

CHICKEN PIZZA

Do you think lactose-intolerant IBD patients cannot eat pizza anymore? You might be wrong! Try this recipe to have a great pizza taste!

- Prep Time: 10 minutes
- Cook Time: 15 minutes

- Total Time: 25 minutes
- Serving: 4

Ingredients

- 4 gluten-free pizza crusts
- 1 cup sliced no-fat cooked chicken breast
- 1 cup shredded mozzarella or lactose-free cheese
- 4 tablespoons organic mayonnaise
- 1 teaspoon oregano powder

Instructions

1. Place your gluten-free pizza crusts on a non-stick pizza pan or bake sheet.
2. Spread your organic low-fat low-sodium mayo on your crust.
3. Add your cooked chicken breasts to your pizza
4. Sprinkle with mozzarella or lactose-free cheese
5. Let it bake at 480 °F for 10 minutes. Then, broil on the same heat for five more minutes until cheese melted.

Cooking Tips:

- You can use any other white sauces such as béchamel sauce instead of mayo.

Low residue diet-related Tips:

- If you are lactose intolerant, use lactose-free or dairy-free cheese for pizza
- Use mayonnaise only if you can tolerate it. If you cannot tolerate, you can make a béchamel sauce instead (explained before in Fettuccine Alfredo recipe).

Nutrition Facts	
Servings: 4	
Amount per serving	
Calories	**342**
	% Daily Value*
Total Fat 12.4g	16%
Saturated Fat 2.7g	14%
Cholesterol 47mg	16%
Sodium 499mg	22%
Total Carbohydrate 39.1g	14%
Dietary Fiber 2.1g	7%
Total Sugars 7g	
Protein 18.5g	
Vitamin D 0mcg	0%
Calcium 82mg	6%
Iron 1mg	7%
Potassium 165mg	4%

TURKEY ZUCCHINI NOODLES

If you look for a healthy meal for your lunch or dinner, you can try Turkey Zucchini Noodles. If you have some leftover turkeys from Thanksgiving or any other events, it would be an excellent option for you to cook this delicious main course.

- Prep Time: 15 minutes
- Cook Time: 15 minutes
- Total Time: 30 minutes
- Serving: 4

Ingredients

- 3 medium-size spiralized zucchinis or zucchini strips
- 1 lb (~455 g) skinless fat-free cooked turkey breasts
- 1 tablespoon extra virgin olive oil, divided
- 2 cups of water
- ½ teaspoon turmeric
- ½ teaspoon salt
- 1 tablespoon tomato paste (optional)
- ¼ teaspoon stevia (optional)

Instructions

1. Cook zucchini noodles in boiling water for 5 minutes.
2. Bring them out of the water and let them dry.
3. Heat your cooked turkey in a pan with extra virgin olive oil. Add turmeric, tomato paste (optional), stevia (optional) salt, and little water (~100ml) for 5 minutes until golden brown both sides.
4. Add your zucchini to your turkey and stir well. Enjoy!

Cooking Tips:

- You can use a can of organic crushed tomatoes instead of tomato paste if you can tolerate them.

Low residue diet-related Tips:

- If you are in a flare-up, do not need to golden-brown turkey. Just boil it in 1 cup of zucchini water.

Nutrition Facts
Servings: 4

Amount per serving	
Calories	**172**
	% Daily Value*
Total Fat 5.7g	7%
Saturated Fat 0.9g	5%
Cholesterol 49mg	16%
Sodium 1460mg	63%
Total Carbohydrate 9.9g	4%
Dietary Fiber 2.3g	8%
Total Sugars 6.5g	
Protein 21.2g	
Vitamin D 0mcg	0%
Calcium 35mg	3%
Iron 2mg	13%
Potassium 736mg	16%

Zucchini Egg Dish

Are you looking for a vegetarian dish that is well-matched with low residue diet patient's diet? Try a fabulous Zucchini Egg dish.

- Prep Time: 10 minutes

- Cook Time: 15 minutes
- Total Time: 25 minutes
- Serving: 4

Ingredients

- 3 medium-size, diced zucchinis
- 2 organic range-free eggs
- 1 tablespoon extra virgin olive oil
- ½ teaspoon turmeric powder
- ½ teaspoon salt
- ½ teaspoon black pepper

Instructions

1. Peels off zucchinis and cook them in a pan over medium heat.
2. When zucchinis become soft, flattened them or blend them in a blender.
3. Add turmeric, salt, and pepper to your pan.
4. Whisk eggs in a small bowl and add them to your zucchinis.
5. When the eggs get coagulate, mix them with your zucchinis. Enjoy!

Cooking Tips:

- You can use eggplant instead of zucchini.
- You can also add one tablespoon of tomato paste if you can tolerate it.

Low residue diet-related Tips:

- If you are in a flare-up, do not need to fry zucchinis. Just boil them in 1 cup of water.

- Do not use black pepper in your meal if you are in a severe flare-up.

Nutrition Facts
Servings: 4

Amount per serving	
Calories	**94**
	% Daily Value*
Total Fat 6g	8%
Saturated Fat 1.2g	6%
Cholesterol 82mg	27%
Sodium 337mg	15%
Total Carbohydrate 7g	3%
Dietary Fiber 2g	7%
Total Sugars 3.2g	
Protein 5g	
Vitamin D 8mcg	39%
Calcium 37mg	3%
Iron 1mg	7%
Potassium 448mg	10%

Potato Cutlet

Potato Cutlet is an easy to cook vegetarian recipe for IBD patients with a yummy crispy texture.

- Prep Time: 10 minutes
- Cook Time: 20 minutes
- Total Time: 30 minutes
- Serving: 4

Ingredients

- 2 lbs yellow skin-removed potatoes
- 5 large organic range-free eggs
- 3 tablespoons extra virgin olive oil
- ½ teaspoon turmeric powder
- Salt and black pepper to taste

Instructions

1. Remove potato skins and scrub potatoes with a scrubber.

2. In a large bowl, mix potatoes and all other ingredients perfectly.
3. Make potato cutlets by rounding-and-flattening them in your hand.
4. Heat your high-quality extra virgin olive oil in a skillet over medium heat. Add your cutlets to the pan and flatten them.
5. Let it cook each side until golden brown.

Cooking Tips:

- You can add one teaspoon freshly grated ginger to your ingredients, as well.

Low residue diet-related Tips:

- If you are in a flare-up, do not need to fry potatoes. Just boil them in water and then mix them with other ingredients.
- Do not use black pepper in your meal if you are in a severe flare-up.

Nutrition Facts	
Servings: 4	
Amount per serving	
Calories	**273**
	% Daily Value*
Total Fat 10.6g	14%
Saturated Fat 1.5g	8%
Cholesterol 0mg	0%
Sodium 112mg	5%
Total Carbohydrate 40.5g	15%
Dietary Fiber 4.1g	15%
Total Sugars 2.3g	
Protein 8.5g	
Vitamin D 0mcg	0%
Calcium 164mg	13%
Iron 2mg	13%
Potassium 75mg	2%

GINGER STICKY PORK

Are you looking for a satisfying, easy to cook a meal with pork? Ginger Sticky Pork is a great candidate for you and your family members who is on a low residue diet.

- Prep Time: 15 minutes
- Cook Time: 10 minutes
- Total Time: 25 minutes
- Serving: 6

Ingredients

- 1½ lb boneless, fat-removed pork tenderloin, cut into strips with ½ inch (~1.3cm) thickness
- 1 tablespoon extra virgin olive oil
- ½ cup honey or maple syrup
- 2 inches (~5cm) fresh ginger knob
- 1 tablespoon lemon juice
- 1 teaspoon salt
- ½ teaspoon black pepper

Instructions

1. Heat extra virgin olive oil in a skillet over medium-high heat until shimmering.
2. Add your pork, salt, and pepper to the skillet. Brown one side first and then brown the other side of pork. Take out your pork.
3. Add ginger, lemon juice, and honey to the pan. Stir and bring to boil.
4. When the sauce gets thick and sticky like honey, bring back your pork. Enjoy!

Cooking Tips:

- This dish can be served perfectly with white steamed rice.

Low residue diet-related Tips:

- Boil pork in water if you are in a severe flare-up. Then, take the pork out of boiling water and add them to your sticky sauce.
- If you cannot use honey, you can use maple syrup, ½ teaspoon of stevia or agave syrup.
- Do not use black pepper in your meal if you are in a severe flare-up.

Nutrition Facts	
Servings: 6	
Amount per serving	
Calories	**275**
	% Daily Value*
Total Fat 6.4g	8%
Saturated Fat 1.7g	9%
Cholesterol 83mg	28%
Sodium 454mg	20%
Total Carbohydrate 24.9g	9%
Dietary Fiber 0.4g	1%
Total Sugars 23.5g	
Protein 30g	
Vitamin D 0mcg	0%
Calcium 12mg	1%
Iron 2mg	9%
Potassium 521mg	11%

German Pork Schnitzel

If you are looking for tender pork with a crispy crust, try German Pork Schnitzel. It is very easy to make it, and it is well-matched with baby carrots and potato garnishes.

- Prep Time: 20 minutes
- Cook Time: 15 minutes
- Total Time: 35 minutes
- Serving: 4

Ingredients

- 2 lbs boneless fatless pork tenderloins flattened into ½ inch (1.3cm) thick

- 3 large organic free-range eggs
- 2 cups bread crumbs or gluten-free bread crumbs
- ⅓ cup all-purpose flour or gluten-free flour
- 2 tablespoons extra virgin olive oil
- Lemon wedges for taste
- ½ teaspoon salt
- ½ teaspoon black pepper

Instructions

1. Pound your pork pieces with a mallet until it gets ½ inch thick.
2. In a medium bowl, mix flour, and pepper.
3. In another bowl, whisk three eggs.
4. In another bowl or plate, spread your breadcrumbs.
5. First, put both sides of pork cutlets in flour. Then, dip them in egg and then drip them into breadcrumbs using a fork.
6. Now, heat a large pan with extra virgin olive oil over medium heat. When the oil gets very hot, cook your cutlets for 5 minutes, each side until each side gets golden brown.
7. Enjoy the meal with lemon wedges!

Cooking Tips:

- This dish can be served perfectly with mashed potatoes. If you are lactose-intolerant, use lactose-free milk to make mashed potatoes.
- Use gluten-free bread crumbs and flour if you are gluten intolerant.

Low residue diet-related Tips:

- Do not use black pepper in your meal if you are in a severe flare-up.
- Use only one egg if you cannot tolerate eggs well during a flare-up.

Nutrition Facts	
Servings: 4	
Amount per serving	
Calories	**600**
	% Daily Value*
Total Fat 19.3g	25%
Saturated Fat 4.7g	23%
Cholesterol 243mg	81%
Sodium 979mg	43%
Total Carbohydrate 49.6g	18%
Dietary Fiber 2.9g	10%
Total Sugars 5.7g	
Protein 54.5g	
Vitamin D 12mcg	58%
Calcium 120mg	9%
Iron 6mg	33%
Potassium 169mg	4%

Baked Apple Pork

A delicious pork-based recipe that has been modified for IBD patients.

- Prep Time: 5 minutes
- Cook Time: 35 minutes
- Total Time: 40 minutes
- Serving: 4

<u>Ingredients</u>

- 2 lbs skinless, boneless pork tenderloin
- 1 cup large apple, cut into small cubes
- 1 tablespoon peeled and grated ginger (~1 inch or ~2.5 cm)
- 2 tablespoons soy sauce
- 2 tablespoons extra virgin olive oil
- Salt and black pepper to taste

Instructions

1. Mix ginger, balsamic, and soy sauce in a small bowl.
2. Add salt and pepper to your pork.
3. Use a large skillet and cook both sides of your pork in it over medium heat with high-quality extra virgin olive oil until golden brown.
4. Check by a knife to see if the inside pork cooked or not. Remove the pork pieces from the skillet. Add your sauce to the pan and let it cooked for three more minutes.
5. Poach your apple in for 15 minutes in boiling water.
6. Bring back pork pieces to the skillet and let it cook for one more minute.

Cooking Tips:

- This dish can be served with steamed white rice.

Low residue diet-related Tips:

- Do not use black pepper if you are experiencing a severe flare-up.

Nutrition Facts

Servings: 4

Amount per serving

Calories 375

	% Daily Value*
Total Fat 15.2g	19%
Saturated Fat 4g	20%
Cholesterol 132mg	44%
Sodium 533mg	23%
Total Carbohydrate 7.4g	3%
Dietary Fiber 0.7g	2%
Total Sugars 5.5g	
Protein 51.3g	
Vitamin D 0mcg	0%
Calcium 7mg	1%
Iron 2mg	10%
Potassium 68mg	1%

BALSAMIC-PEACH PORK

Balsamic-Peach Pork is a great and easy-to-cook meal with few ingredients. A fantastic combination of peach and honey gives the dish a lovely sweet taste.

- Prep Time: 10 minutes
- Cook Time: 20 minutes
- Total Time: 30 minutes
- Serving: 4

Ingredients

- 2 boneless pork tenderloins
- 2 sliced peeled peaches
- 6 oz low-fat feta cheese or lactose-free Swiss cheese
- 1 tablespoon honey or maple syrup
- 2 tablespoons extra virgin olive oil
- 1 tablespoon fresh chopped oregano or thyme leaves
- Salt and black pepper to taste
- ½ cup fresh basil (optional)

Instructions

1. Mix cheese, honey (or maple syrup), oregano, or thyme leaves in a bowl.
2. Add salt and pepper to your pork.
3. Use a large skillet and cook both sides of your pork in it over medium heat with high-quality extra virgin olive oil until golden brown.
4. Check by knife if inside pork cooked well. Remove the pork pieces from the skillet. Add your sauce to the pan and let it cooked for three more minutes.
5. Cook your peeled-off peaches in the same skillet for five minutes. If your sauce gets dry, add water a little bit.

6. Bring back pork pieces to the skillet and let it cook for two more minutes.
7. Garnish with fresh basil if you want. Enjoy!

Cooking Tips:

- This dish can be served well with steamed white rice.
- You can have lactose-free Havarti cheese instead of low-fat feta or Swiss cheese.

Low residue diet-related Tips:

- Do not use black pepper or many green basils if you are experiencing a severe flare-up.
- If you cannot tolerate honey, remove honey from your recipe or use one tablespoon of stevia instead.

Nutrition Facts
Servings: 4

Amount per serving	
Calories	**266**
	% Daily Value*
Total Fat 15.6g	20%
Saturated Fat 1.5g	8%
Cholesterol 31mg	10%
Sodium 476mg	21%
Total Carbohydrate 14.6g	5%
Dietary Fiber 1.7g	6%
Total Sugars 11.5g	
Protein 18.7g	
Vitamin D 1mcg	6%
Calcium 585mg	45%
Iron 2mg	11%
Potassium 355mg	8%

Honey-Turmeric Pork

If you are looking for a healthy dish, you are reading the right recipe. A short cooking-time Honey-Turmeric Pork is an excellent choice for IBD patients who wants to have a rich pork-based main course.

- Prep Time: 15 minutes

- Cook Time: 15 minutes
- Total Time: 30 minutes
- Serving: 4

Ingredients

- 1¼ pounds chopped boneless, fat-removed pork tenderloin
- ½ cup plain yogurt or plain lactose-free yogurt
- ¼ cup honey or maple syrup
- 2 tablespoons extra virgin olive oil
- 3 small carrots
- 1½ teaspoons turmeric powder
- 3 tablespoons fresh lemon juice
- Salt and black pepper to taste
- 3 small beets, sliced thin (optional)

Instructions

1. Mix plain yogurt, honey (or maple syrup), turmeric, and lemon juice in a bowl.
2. Pour salt and pepper on your pork.
3. Use a large skillet and cook both sides of your pork in it over medium heat with high-quality extra virgin olive oil until golden brown.
4. Check by knife if inside pork cooked well. Remove the pork pieces from the skillet. Add your sauce to the pan and let it cooked for three more minutes.
5. Cook your peeled-off beets (optional) and carrots in a small skillet for 10 minutes as sides.
6. Bring back pork pieces to the skillet and let it cook for two more minutes. Enjoy it with carrot and beet sides!

Cooking Tips:

- This dish can be served well with steamed white rice or noodles.
- If you are lactose-intolerant, use lactose-free plain yogurt or remove yogurt from the recipe.

Low residue diet-related Tips:

- Do not use black pepper or beets if you are experiencing a severe flare-up.
- If you cannot tolerate honey, remove honey from your recipe or use one tablespoon of stevia instead.

Nutrition Facts
Servings: 4

Amount per serving	
Calories	**624**
	% Daily Value*
Total Fat 18.7g	24%
Saturated Fat 5.2g	26%
Cholesterol 229mg	76%
Sodium 235mg	10%
Total Carbohydrate 26.4g	10%
Dietary Fiber 1.9g	7%
Total Sugars 22.2g	
Protein 84.1g	
Vitamin D 0mcg	0%
Calcium 98mg	8%
Iron 5mg	28%
Potassium 1633mg	35%

GRILLED LEAN BEEF KEBAB

IBD patients have to significantly reduce red meat in their diet as typically, red meat meals are harder to digest, and they can cause flare-ups. Extra-lean beef with no fats is recommended for IBD patients who want to consume red meats. Another fabulous alternative to red meat is Ostrich meat. It tastes very similar to lean beef, but it has less fat, cholesterol. It is high in calcium, iron, and protein. It is highly recommended for IBD patients to include Ostrich beef in their diet once a week.

- Prep Time: 10 minutes

- Marinate Time: 60 minutes
- Cook Time: 20 minutes
- Total Time: 90 minutes
- Serving: 4

Ingredients

- 2 lbs extra lean beef or lamb meat
- ½ cup plain yogurt or plain lactose-free yogurt
- 1 small kiwi
- 1 onion (thinly sliced)
- 1 tablespoon extra virgin olive oil
- 4 tablespoons fresh lemon juice
- Salt and black pepper to taste

Instructions

1. Cut extra lean beef/lamb into small 1-inch (~2.54cm) cubes.
2. Ina large bowl, marinate your beef/lamb with plain yogurt, onion, kiwi, lemon juice, olive oil, salt, and pepper.
3. Cover the top bowl, fridge it and Let it marinate for 1 hour.
4. Skewer your kebab cubes or just grill both sides like a steak. Ten minutes grill would suffice for medium kebabs, and 20 minutes grill would suffice for well-done kebabs.

Cooking Tips:

- You do not necessarily need to cut your beef/lamb into cubes. You can flatten them by mallet and make a fantastic steak.
- Kiwi melts your kebab and makes it very juicy.

- This dish can be served well with steamed white rice.
- If you are lactose-intolerant, use lactose-free plain yogurt or remove yogurt from the recipe.

Low residue diet-related Tips:

- Do not use black pepper or onion if you are experiencing a severe flare-up.

Nutrition Facts	
Servings: 4	
Amount per serving	
Calories	**499**
	% Daily Value*
Total Fat 18.3g	23%
Saturated Fat 6.3g	31%
Cholesterol 205mg	68%
Sodium 176mg	8%
Total Carbohydrate 7.9g	3%
Dietary Fiber 1.2g	4%
Total Sugars 5.4g	
Protein 71.2g	
Vitamin D 0mcg	0%
Calcium 73mg	6%
Iron 43mg	238%
Potassium 1104mg	23%

HUNGARIAN GOULASH

Goulash is a great traditional stew full of healthy ingredients. IBD patients need to add more bone, beef, chicken, or vegetable broth meals in their diet. Hungarian Goulash is a great option that can be added to your weekly meal plan.

- Prep Time: 30 minutes
- Cook Time: 90 minutes
- Total Time: 120 minutes
- Serving: 6

Ingredients

- 1½ lbs extra lean beef trimmed into 1 inch (~2.54 cm) cubes
- 2 cups bone/beef broth or tap water
- 2 tablespoons extra virgin olive oil
- 2 tablespoons lemon juice
- ½ tablespoon turmeric
- 1 teaspoon salt
- ¼ teaspoon pepper
- 1 cup carrots
- 2 cups potatoes, cut into 1 inch (~2.54cm) cubes
- 1 tablespoon tomato paste (optional)

Instructions

1. One a large pan or a pot, heat olive oil, turmeric, tomato paste (optional), and pepper over medium heat.
2. Add your extra lean beef and stir for 5 minutes.
3. Add water or bone/beef broth slowly to your pot. Then, cover and let it cook for 50 minutes over low heat until tender.
4. Add potatoes and let it cook for 20 more minutes. Add salt and lemon juice. Then, add the carrots and cook the stew for 15 more minutes. Enjoy!

Cooking Tips:

- This dish can be served well with steamed white rice.
- Anytime the stew gets very thick, add more water into it.

Low residue diet-related Tips:

- Do not use black pepper or tomato paste if you are experiencing a severe flare-up.

Nutrition Facts	
Servings: 6	
Amount per serving	
Calories	309
	% Daily Value*
Total Fat 12.4g	16%
Saturated Fat 3.5g	18%
Cholesterol 101mg	34%
Sodium 734mg	32%
Total Carbohydrate 10.5g	4%
Dietary Fiber 1.8g	6%
Total Sugars 1.8g	
Protein 37.1g	
Vitamin D 0mcg	0%
Calcium 17mg	1%
Iron 22mg	123%
Potassium 810mg	17%

Tomato Free Spaghetti Bolognese

Many of IBD patients cannot well-tolerated tomatoes and tomato pastes, which can negatively affect their regular cooking habits using tomatoes inside meals. Let us try a great Spaghetti Bolognese tomato-free! Yes, you read correctly! Enjoy a tomato-free Italian dish now!

- Prep Time: 15 minutes
- Cook Time: 25 minutes
- Total Time: 40 minutes
- Serving: 4

Ingredients

- 1 lb (~500 s) extra lean ground beef
- 0.65 lb (~300 g) spaghetti or gluten-free spaghetti
- 1 cup organic unsalted chicken stock
- 1 tablespoon extra virgin olive oil
- 1 tablespoon soy sauce
- 2 tablespoons maple syrup
- 1 teaspoon dried oregano or oregano powder
- ½ teaspoon dried thyme
- 1 teaspoon dried basil

- ½ tablespoon turmeric
- 1 teaspoon salt
- ¼ teaspoon pepper
- 1 tablespoon of Parmesan or any lactose-free cheese (optional)

Instructions

1. Golden both sides of your extra lean ground beef in a large pan with extra virgin olive oil over high heat.
2. Add soy sauce, honey (or maple syrup), salt, pepper, turmeric, and chicken stock to your ground beef. Let it thicken and have it cooked for one more minute.
3. At the same time, prepare your spaghetti according to its package recipe with a pinch of salt and a little bit of olive oil.
4. Take your spaghetti out of boiling water and put it in your sauce.
5. Season it with dried basil.

Cooking Tips:

- You can add some lactose-free cheese to this recipe if you are lactose intolerant.
- If your sauce thickened more than desired, add some tap water or spaghetti boiling water.

Low residue diet-related Tips:

- Do not use black pepper, Parmesan, or fresh herbs if you are experiencing a severe flare-up.

Nutrition Facts	
Servings: 4	
Amount per serving	
Calories	**475**
	% Daily Value*
Total Fat 12.9g	17%
Saturated Fat 4.2g	21%
Cholesterol 141mg	47%
Sodium 1092mg	47%
Total Carbohydrate 49.1g	18%
Dietary Fiber 0.5g	2%
Total Sugars 6.3g	
Protein 38.8g	
Vitamin D 0mcg	0%
Calcium 42mg	3%
Iron 7mg	37%
Potassium 593mg	13%

Lamb/Beef Liver stew

A great stew with excellent sources of Iron, Vitamin A, D, and B12 for IBD patients. However, the lamb/beef liver has to be used with caution in patients who have high cholesterol.

- Prep Time: 10 minutes
- Cook Time: 20 minutes
- Total Time: 30 minutes
- Serving: 4

Ingredients

- 1 lb (~500 g) lamb/beef liver, cut in 1 inch (~2.54cm) cubes
- 1 cup of organic unsalted bone/beef broth
- 2 tablespoons extra virgin olive oil
- 2 teaspoons turmeric
- 1 teaspoon salt
- ½ teaspoon pepper
- 1 potato, cut into 1 inch (~2.54cm) cubes (optional)
- 2 tablespoons tomato paste (optional)

Instructions

1. Fully cook your lamb/beef liver in a large pan with extra virgin olive oil, turmeric, salt and pepper, potatoes (optional), and tomato paste (optional) over medium heat for 15 minutes.
2. Add your bone/beef broth to your livers. Cook for 5 minutes until thickened.

Cooking Tips:

- You can add 1 tablespoon of flour or gluten-free flour if your stew is not getting thick.
- If your stew thickened more than desired, add some hot water to it.

Low residue diet-related Tips:

- Do not use black pepper and tomato paste if you are experiencing a flare-up.
- If you are in high cholesterol, you can substitute the liver with the extra lean ostrich.

Nutrition Facts
Servings: 4

Amount per serving

Calories	273
	% Daily Value*
Total Fat 12.8g	16%
Saturated Fat 2.8g	14%
Cholesterol 432mg	144%
Sodium 860mg	37%
Total Carbohydrate 7g	3%
Dietary Fiber 0.3g	1%
Total Sugars 0.2g	
Protein 31.4g	
Vitamin D 0mcg	0%
Calcium 13mg	1%
Iron 8mg	43%
Potassium 481mg	10%

GRILLED HONEY SALMON

Try a yummy grilled honey salmon dish. Those who are in a severe flare-up, can your maple syrup in moderation instead of honey.

- Prep Time: 5 minutes
- Cook Time: 25 minutes
- Total Time: 30 minutes
- Serving: 4

Ingredients:

- 2 lbs (~1 kg) salmon fillets
- ¼ cup honey or maple syrup
- 1 tablespoon extra virgin olive oil
- 1 teaspoon turmeric powder
- 1 tablespoon fresh thyme leaves
- Salt and black pepper, to taste

Directions:

1. Choose a medium bowl and whisk honey (or maple syrup), turmeric, thyme leaves, extra virgin olive oil, salt, and pepper together.
2. Preheat your oven to 375 °F.
3. Pour your sauce over the salmon.
4. Put your salmon in the oven and let it cook for 20 minutes (until inside cooks well).
5. Enjoy!

Cooking Tips:

- If your salmon is thicker, you have to increase the cooking time until inside cooks well.

- You can cover your salmon with foil for having a juicy texture.

Low residue diet-related Tips:

- Do not use black pepper in your meal if you are experiencing a flare-up.
- If you cannot tolerate honey, try maple syrup, agave syrup or a teaspoon of stevia.

Nutrition Facts	
Servings: 4	
Amount per serving	
Calories	**398**
	% Daily Value*
Total Fat 17.6g	23%
Saturated Fat 2.5g	13%
Cholesterol 100mg	33%
Sodium 101mg	4%
Total Carbohydrate 18.3g	7%
Dietary Fiber 0.4g	2%
Total Sugars 17.4g	
Protein 44.2g	
Vitamin D 0mcg	0%
Calcium 95mg	7%
Iron 3mg	15%
Potassium 902mg	19%

OVEN-BASED SALMON AND POTATO

A great mix of salmon and oven-baked potatoes give you a joyful lunch or dinner meal!

- Prep Time: 5 minutes
- Cook Time: 25 minutes
- Total Time: 30 minutes
- Serving: 4

Ingredients

- 4 salmon filets, about 6 ounces each
- 2 medium potatoes, sliced into very thin chips
- 3 tablespoons extra-virgin olive oil, divided

- 2 oranges
- 2 lemons
- Salt and pepper to taste

Instructions

1. Choose a small bowl and whisk orange juice, lemon juice, 1 tablespoon of extra virgin olive oil, salt, and pepper all together to have a juicy sauce.
2. Marinate your salmon with the sauce.
3. Slice potatoes very thin. Drizzle potatoes with two tablespoons of extra virgin olive oil and a pinch of salt.
4. Preheat your oven to 375 °F.
5. Choose a long foil sheet, put potatoes first, and fill the top with your salmon. Close your foil and let the salmon cook for about 25 minutes until inside cooks well.
6. Enjoy!

Cooking Tips:

- If your salmon is very thick, you have to increase the cooking time until inside cooks well.
- Check both salmon and your potato to be cooked. If required, return your salmon and potato to the over for five more minutes until perfection.

Low residue diet-related Tips:

- Do not use black pepper in your meal if you are experiencing a flare-up.
- If you cannot tolerate orange juice, remove it from the recipe.

Nutrition Facts	
Servings: 4	
Amount per serving	
Calories	**443**
	% Daily Value*
Total Fat 21.8g	28%
Saturated Fat 3.1g	16%
Cholesterol 78mg	26%
Sodium 84mg	4%
Total Carbohydrate 28.4g	10%
Dietary Fiber 4.9g	18%
Total Sugars 10g	
Protein 37.4g	
Vitamin D 0mcg	0%
Calcium 117mg	9%
Iron 2mg	11%
Potassium 1248mg	27%

LEMON STEAMED HALIBUT WITH WHITE RICE

A great dish with healthy ingredients for IBD patients. You can substitute halibut with any other fishes you would like to have.

- Prep Time: 10 minutes
- Cook Time: 30 minutes
- Total Time: 40 minutes
- Serving: 6

<u>Ingredients</u>

- 6 skinless and boneless halibut fillets, about 6 ounces each
- 2 cups steamed white rice
- 1 tablespoon extra virgin olive oil
- 1 lemon, sliced very thin
- 4 tablespoons lemon juice
- 1 teaspoon ginger powder
- Salt and pepper to taste
- Lemon wedges to garnish

<u>Instructions</u>

1. Choose a small bowl and whisk lemon juice, ginger powder, extra virgin olive oil, salt, and pepper all together to have a juicy sauce.
2. Marinate your halibut with the sauce.
3. Preheat your oven to 375 °F.
4. Choose a long foil sheet, put halibut in your foil sheet, and close it. Let it cook for about 25 minutes until inside cooks well.
5. Open the foil sheet, put thin lemon slices on top of your halibut for 5 minutes, and close the foil sheet again.
6. Steam your white rice. Open your foil sheet and put halibut on top of the rice.
7. Garnish with lemon wedges. Enjoy!

Cooking Tips:

- If your halibut is very thick, you have to increase the cooking time until inside cooks well.

Low residue diet-related Tips:

- Do not use black pepper in your meal if you are experiencing a flare-up.

Nutrition Facts
Servings: 6

Amount per serving	
Calories	**568**
	% Daily Value*
Total Fat 9.5g	12%
Saturated Fat 1.4g	7%
Cholesterol 93mg	31%
Sodium 161mg	7%
Total Carbohydrate 50.2g	18%
Dietary Fiber 1.3g	4%
Total Sugars 0.3g	
Protein 65g	
Vitamin D 0mcg	0%
Calcium 33mg	3%
Iron 16mg	87%
Potassium 1396mg	30%

Thunfisch Pizza

Thunfisch Pizza is an excellent German-based pizza with Tuna. The classic recipe has been modified to be tolerated by most IBD patients.

- Prep Time: 5 minutes
- Cook Time: 15 minutes
- Total Time: 20 minutes
- Serving: 4

Ingredients

- 2 medium-size gluten-free pizza crusts
- 1 cup shredded mozzarella or lactose-free cheese pizza
- Two 6.5 oz tuna can on oil or water
- 2 tablespoons organic mayonnaise
- 2 teaspoons dried ground oregano
- Salt to taste

Instructions

1. Place your gluten-free pizza crusts on a non-stick pizza pan or bake sheet.
2. Spread your organic mayo on your crust.
3. Gently put tuna on your pizza crust.
4. Sprinkle with mozzarella or lactose-free cheese
5. Let it bake at 400 °F for 10 minutes. Then, broil on the same heat for five more minutes until cheese melted.

Cooking Tips:

- You can use any other white sauces such as a béchamel sauce (explained before in Fettuccine Alfredo recipe) instead of mayonnaise.

Low residue diet-related Tips:

- If you are lactose intolerant, use lactose-free or dairy-free cheese pizza.
- Use mayonnaise only if you can tolerate it. If you cannot tolerate, you can make a béchamel sauce (explain before in Fettuccine Alfredo recipe) instead.

Nutrition Facts	
Servings: 4	
Amount per serving	
Calories	**297**
	% Daily Value*
Total Fat 13g	17%
Saturated Fat 2.9g	14%
Cholesterol 33mg	11%
Sodium 333mg	14%
Total Carbohydrate 17g	6%
Dietary Fiber 0.8g	3%
Total Sugars 1.5g	
Protein 26.8g	
Vitamin D 0mcg	0%
Calcium 21mg	2%
Iron 1mg	5%
Potassium 310mg	7%

AVOCADO TUNA PITA

A very fast sandwich you can prepare at home for your lunch or dinner. You can even have a smaller portion of avocado tuna as a breakfast or as a snack at work.

- Prep Time: 10 minutes
- Cook Time: 0 minutes
- Total Time: 10 minutes
- Serving: 4

Ingredients

- 2 avocados
- 2 tablespoons organic mayonnaise
- 1 teaspoon cumin powder
- 1 can of tuna in olive oil or water

- ¼ cup apple, chopped and peeled off
- 4 Pita bread or any gluten-free bread
- Salt to taste
- Pepper to taste (optional)

Instructions

1. Choose a small bowl. Mix tuna with smashed avocado with mayo, cumin powder, peeled off apple (cut into small pieces), salt, and pepper (optional).
2. Open each of your pita bread from the corner and spoon the mix inside.
3. Roll the pita. Enjoy!

Cooking Tips:

- You can make this sandwich without mayonnaise sauce, as well.

Low residue diet-related Tips:

- Do not use black pepper or cumin powder, if you are experiencing a flare-up.

Nutrition Facts

Servings: 4

Amount per serving

Calories	491
	% Daily Value*
Total Fat 26.5g	34%
Saturated Fat 5.3g	27%
Cholesterol 16mg	5%
Sodium 442mg	19%
Total Carbohydrate 46g	17%
Dietary Fiber 8.5g	30%
Total Sugars 3.2g	
Protein 19.4g	
Vitamin D 0mcg	0%
Calcium 71mg	5%
Iron 3mg	16%
Potassium 733mg	16%

TROUT WITH ORANGE

Great classic seafood that typically serves with steamed white rice. It is recommended to make this dish with bitter or blood oranges.

- Prep Time: 20 minutes
- Cook Time: 30 minutes
- Total Time: 50 minutes
- Serving: 6

Ingredients

- Large fresh trout, 1.5 lbs each
- 3 oranges
- 1 tablespoon lemon juice
- 1 tablespoon extra virgin olive oil
- ½ teaspoon turmeric powder
- Salt & pepper to taste

Instructions

1. Choose a medium bowl and whisk lemon juice, orange juice, turmeric powder, extra virgin olive oil, salt, and pepper all together to have a juicy sauce.
2. Marinate your trout with the sauce. For better taste, you may need to let it rest at room temperature for 30 minutes.
3. Preheat your oven to 375 °F.
4. Choose a long foil sheet, put trout in your foil sheet and close it. Let it cook for about 25 minutes until inside cooks well.
5. Enjoy!

Cooking Tips:

- Check your trout until inside cooked well. You may need more minutes for perfection.

- This dish can be served with potatoes or steamed white rice.
- You can substitute orange with mango or lemon juice if you like to try other great flavors.

Low residue diet-related Tips:

- Do not use black pepper if you are experiencing a flare-up.

Nutrition Facts	
Servings: 4	
Amount per serving	
Calories	**391**
	% Daily Value*
Total Fat 16.9g	22%
Saturated Fat 2.8g	14%
Cholesterol 115mg	38%
Sodium 105mg	5%
Total Carbohydrate 16.5g	6%
Dietary Fiber 3.4g	12%
Total Sugars 13g	
Protein 42.6g	
Vitamin D 0mcg	0%
Calcium 141mg	11%
Iron 3mg	18%
Potassium 980mg	21%

CHICKEN AND SHRIMP TERIYAKI

A lovely Edo-style mix of chicken and shrimp with healthy ingredients for IBD patients.

- Prep Time: 5 minutes
- Cook Time: 20 minutes
- Total Time: 25 minutes
- Serving: 4

Ingredients

- 2 lbs (~1 kg) organic chicken breast, chopped in cubes
- 24 shrimps, peeled and deveined

- 1 tablespoon ginger powder, divided
- 2 tablespoons extra virgin olive oil
- ½ teaspoon turmeric
- ⅓ cup gluten-free and sodium-reduced soy sauce
- ⅓ cup of cold water
- 3 teaspoons arrowroot powder
- ¼ cup honey, or maple syrup
- Salt & pepper to taste

Instructions

1. In a medium bowl, whisk ginger powder, one tablespoon of olive oil, soy sauce, arrowroot powder, honey (or maple syrup), water, salt, and pepper to make a juicy teriyaki sauce.
2. Let Teriyaki sauce rest in the fridge for 5 minutes.
3. In a large pan, add one tablespoon of olive oil and cook chicken over medium heat until golden brown both sides.
4. Add your sauce and shrimp to the pan. Stir and mix for 5 minutes until thickened.
5. Enjoy!

Cooking Tips:

- You can serve this dish with steamed white rice or rice noodles.

Low residue diet-related Tips:

- Do not use black pepper if you are experiencing a severe flare-up.
- Use maple syrup or stevia (1 teaspoon) if you cannot tolerate honey.

Nutrition Facts	
Servings: 4	
Amount per serving	
Calories	**553**
	% Daily Value*
Total Fat 15.1g	19%
Saturated Fat 1.7g	9%
Cholesterol 423mg	141%
Sodium 1639mg	71%
Total Carbohydrate 20g	7%
Dietary Fiber 0.4g	1%
Total Sugars 12.1g	
Protein 79.6g	
Vitamin D 0mcg	1%
Calcium 151mg	12%
Iron 2mg	12%
Potassium 1175mg	25%

LEMON SHRIMP WITH WHITE RICE

Lemon Shrimp with steamed white rice is very easy to make and a healthy dish you can have in your weekly diet.

- Prep Time: 5 minutes
- Cook Time: 20 minutes
- Total Time: 25 minutes
- Serving: 4

Ingredients

- 24 shrimps, peeled and deveined
- 2 tablespoons extra virgin olive oil, divided
- ½ teaspoon turmeric powder
- 4 tablespoons lemon juice
- 3 cups of white rice
- 1 teaspoon salt & pepper

Instructions

1. In a small bowl, whisk lemon juice, one tablespoon of olive oil, turmeric powder, salt, and pepper to make a sauce.
2. Cook your rice according to its package instructions.

3. Add one tablespoon of high-quality extra virgin olive oil in a pan and cook shrimp over medium heat for 5-7 minutes.
4. Add your sauce into the pan. Stir and mix well for 5 minutes.
5. Enjoy!

Cooking Tips:

- You can serve the lemon shrimp with rice noodles instead of white rice.

Low residue diet-related Tips:

- Do not use black pepper if you are experiencing a severe flare-up.

Nutrition Facts

Servings: 4

Amount per serving	
Calories	**729**
	% Daily Value*
Total Fat 10.3g	13%
Saturated Fat 2.1g	10%
Cholesterol 278mg	93%
Sodium 332mg	14%
Total Carbohydrate 113.8g	41%
Dietary Fiber 2.1g	7%
Total Sugars 0.5g	
Protein 40.2g	
Vitamin D 0mcg	0%
Calcium 162mg	12%
Iron 7mg	37%
Potassium 416mg	9%

HONEY PRAWN LINGUINE

Are you looking for an Italian seafood linguine recipe for IBD patients? You have to try this delicious main course.

- Prep Time: 5 minutes
- Cook Time: 20 minutes
- Total Time: 25 minutes

- Serving: 4

Ingredients:

- 1 lb (~500 gr) prawns, peeled and deveined
- 1 lb (~500 gr) cooked linguine or any gluten-free pasta
- 2 tablespoons extra virgin olive oil, divided
- 4 tablespoons honey or maple syrup
- ½ cup carrot
- ½ cup of water
- Salt and black pepper to taste
- ¼ cup green onion (only if tolerated)

Instructions

1. Whisk honey (or maple syrup), one tablespoon of olive oil, carrot, green onion, pepper, and salt in a proper bowl to make a sauce.
2. Cook your linguini according to its package instructions.
3. Add one tablespoon of high-quality extra virgin olive oil in a medium-size pan and cook prawns over medium heat for 5-7 minutes.
4. Add your sauce into the pan. Stir and mix well for 5 minutes until sauce gets thick.
5. Add pasta to your sauce and mix all well. Enjoy!

Cooking Tips:

- You can serve honey prawn linguine with rice noodles or any other kinds of pasta instead of linguini.

Low residue diet-related Tips:

- Do not use black pepper, and green onion, if you are experiencing a severe flare-up.
- You can use maple syrup, agave syrup, or a teaspoon of stevia if you cannot tolerate honey.

Nutrition Facts
Servings: 4

Amount per serving	
Calories	**592**
	% Daily Value*
Total Fat 11.5g	15%
Saturated Fat 2g	10%
Cholesterol 322mg	107%
Sodium 317mg	14%
Total Carbohydrate 82.7g	30%
Dietary Fiber 0.5g	2%
Total Sugars 18g	
Protein 38.9g	
Vitamin D 0mcg	0%
Calcium 128mg	10%
Iron 4mg	24%
Potassium 461mg	10%

DESSERTS

PEAR CAKE SUNDAES

A delicious dessert with pear, cinnamon, and ice cream. Substantially modified to be consumed by IBD patients.

- Prep Time: 15 minutes
- Total Time: 15 minutes
- Serving: 4

Ingredients

- 2 tablespoons extra virgin olive oil
- ¼ cup brown sugar or one tablespoon honey
- 1 cup pear, chopped
- 1-pint lactose-free vanilla ice cream or sorbet
- 1½ cup vanilla loaf pound cake
- 1 tablespoon maple syrup

- ¼ teaspoon cinnamon powder

Instructions

- In a medium skillet, heat extra virgin olive oil over medium heat. Add brown sugar, cinnamon, and honey. Stir well until brown with a soft texture.
- Add pear and let it cook for two-three more minutes. Remove from heat.
- Preheat oven to 375 °F. Bake your cake for about 8-10 minutes until toasted.
- Crumble vanilla loaf pound cake and place it on top of ice cream scoops (or sorbets). Pour maple syrup on top.
- Add pear sauce. Serve and enjoy!

Cooking Tips:

- You can mix the pear sauce with any cold plain or vanilla yogurt instead of ice cream.

Low residue diet-related Tips:

- Always try to consume less sugar. Instead, you can use honey. If you cannot tolerate honey well, you can use maple syrup or stevia.

Nutrition Facts	
Servings: 4	
Amount per serving	
Calories	**213**
	% Daily Value*
Total Fat 10.8g	14%
Saturated Fat 2.6g	13%
Cholesterol 12mg	4%
Sodium 54mg	2%
Total Carbohydrate 29g	11%
Dietary Fiber 0.7g	3%
Total Sugars 23.5g	
Protein 1.4g	
Vitamin D 0mcg	0%
Calcium 41mg	3%
Iron 1mg	3%
Potassium 78mg	2%

Apple-Ginger Sundaes

This summer sundae is based on a great combination of apple, ginger, and ice cream.

- Prep Time: 20 minutes
- Total Time: 20 minutes
- Serving: 4

Ingredients

- 2 apples, peeled and sliced
- 2 tablespoons extra virgin olive oil
- 2 tablespoons brown sugar or two tablespoon honey
- 6 tablespoons organic no added sugar, apple juice
- ½ teaspoon cornstarch
- 2 cup lactose-free vanilla ice cream or sorbet
- ¼ teaspoon freshly grated ginger

Instructions

- In a large skillet, heat extra virgin olive oil over medium heat. Add apple and ginger and cook for three minutes until tender. Add brown sugar or honey and stir well for 1-2 minutes.

- In a bowl, mix cornstarch and apple juice and pour the mix into the skillet. Cook all mix until thickened.
- Cool for 2-4 minutes.
- Scoop your ice cream or sorbet in a proper dessert plate. Pour your apple ginger mix on top.
- Serve and enjoy!

Cooking Tips:

- You can mix the apple ginger sauce with any cold plain or vanilla yogurt instead of ice cream.

Low residue diet-related Tips:

- Always try to consume less sugar. Instead, you can use honey. If you cannot tolerate honey well, you can use maple syrup or stevia.
- If you cannot tolerate cornstarch well, use all-purpose white flour or rice flour.

Nutrition Facts
Servings: 4

Amount per serving	
Calories	**212**
	% Daily Value*
Total Fat 10.7g	14%
Saturated Fat 3.3g	16%
Cholesterol 10mg	3%
Sodium 20mg	1%
Total Carbohydrate 29.7g	11%
Dietary Fiber 2.7g	10%
Total Sugars 25.2g	
Protein 1.3g	
Vitamin D 0mcg	0%
Calcium 46mg	4%
Iron 1mg	3%
Potassium 151mg	3%

Banana Lemon Trifle

If you want to try a different delicious dessert, you have to make Banana Lemon Trifle.

- Prep Time: 10 minutes
- Total Time: 20 minutes
- Serving: 6

Ingredients

- 4 packs instant vanilla pudding or gluten-free vanilla pudding
- 3 packs shortbread cookies, or gluten-free shortbread cookies
- ½ cup low fat cow milk or almond milk
- 3 bananas, sliced
- 1 tablespoon lemon juice
- Lemon zest
- 4-5 fresh mint leaves

Instructions

- In a large bowl, prepare vanilla pudding according to package instructions. Then mix pudding with lemon juice, lemon zest, and almond milk.
- Top the bowl with shredded shortbread cookies and sliced banana. Garnish with mint leaves.

Cooking Tips:

- You can top the bowl with cinnamon powder as well.

Low residue diet-related Tips:

- Make sure you can tolerate mint leaves. Otherwise, do not use it.
- When in a flare-up, do not use milk. Instead, use boiling water.

Nutrition Facts

Servings: 6

Amount per serving

Calories	481
	% Daily Value*
Total Fat 11.2g	14%
Saturated Fat 6.4g	32%
Cholesterol 28mg	9%
Sodium 1033mg	45%
Total Carbohydrate 94.1g	34%
Dietary Fiber 2.6g	9%
Total Sugars 74.3g	
Protein 2.4g	
Vitamin D 0mcg	0%
Calcium 21mg	2%
Iron 1mg	4%
Potassium 253mg	5%

Warm Apple Crumble

Warm apple crumble is a quick dessert to make for yourself and your family.

- Prep Time: 15 minutes
- Cook Time: 15 minutes
- Total Time: 30 minutes
- Serving: 4

Ingredients

- 2.5 cups apple, peeled and sliced
- 1 teaspoon vanilla extract
- 2 tablespoons sugar or honey
- 1 teaspoon cinnamon powder, divided
- 2 tablespoons extra virgin olive oil
- Lactose-free vanilla ice cream or sorbet (optional)

Instructions

1. In a medium bowl, mix apple, with vanilla, sugar or honey, and half-teaspoon cinnamon powder.
2. Preheat oven to 350 °F.
3. Choose a proper baking dish. Place the mix in it.

4. Bake apples until slightly get golden (about 12-15 minutes).
5. Serve the apple crumble warm (with or without vanilla ice cream or sorbet). Enjoy!

Cooking Tips:

- Your cooking time highly depends on how thin you sliced apples. Keep your eyes on apples to avoid overcooking.

Low residue diet-related Tips:

- Always try to consume less sugar. Instead, you can use honey. If you cannot tolerate honey well, you can use maple syrup or stevia.

Nutrition Facts	
Servings: 4	
Amount per serving	
Calories	177
	% Daily Value*
Total Fat 8.9g	11%
Saturated Fat 2.5g	12%
Cholesterol 0mg	0%
Sodium 2mg	0%
Total Carbohydrate 26.6g	10%
Dietary Fiber 4.1g	15%
Total Sugars 21g	
Protein 0.6g	
Vitamin D 0mcg	0%
Calcium 7mg	1%
Iron 1mg	8%
Potassium 171mg	4%

Apple Quesadillas

If you can tolerate tortilla, then this dessert is an excellent option for you to make. It perfectly comes with ice cream on top.

- Prep Time: 10 minutes
- Cook Time: 10 minutes

- Total Time: 20 minutes
- Serving: 4-6

Ingredients

- 4 pieces of wheat tortillas
- 1 cup old cheddar cheese, shredded
- 1 tablespoon extra virgin olive oil
- 2 large apples, peeled, cored and skin removed
- 2 tablespoons brown sugar or honey
- 4 tablespoons lactose-free ice cream or sorbet

Instructions

1. Preheat oven to 375 °F.
2. Place your tortillas on a proper baking sheet. Sprinkle extra virgin olive oil, and top with cheddar, sugar or honey, and thinly sliced apples on half of each tortilla.
3. Wrap tortilla by folding the other half towards the half with mixture.
4. Bake quesadillas for about 7-10 minutes until golden.
5. Scoop ice cream or sorbet and top it with your apple mix. Enjoy!

Cooking Tips:

- You can use poached apple or warmed canned apple instead. Dice them and top with other ingredients. Cook for 5 minutes.

Low residue diet-related Tips:

- Always try to consume less sugar. Instead, you can use honey. If you cannot tolerate honey well, you can use maple syrup or stevia.

- When in a flare-up, do not have ice cream with your apple quesadillas.

Nutrition Facts
Servings: 6

Amount per serving
Calories 323

	% Daily Value*
Total Fat 19.4g	25%
Saturated Fat 7.7g	38%
Cholesterol 35mg	12%
Sodium 155mg	7%
Total Carbohydrate 31.2g	11%
Dietary Fiber 7.1g	25%
Total Sugars 20g	
Protein 13.4g	
Vitamin D 0mcg	0%
Calcium 56mg	4%
Iron 0mg	2%
Potassium 84mg	2%

Middle-Eastern Rice Pudding

Rice pudding is a well-known dessert everywhere. Try a luxurious taste of new rice pudding for IBD patients!

- Prep Time: 10 minutes
- Cook Time: 30 minutes
- Total Time: 40 minutes
- Serving: 4-6

<u>Ingredients</u>

- 1 cup white rice
- 2 cups low fat milk or lactose-free milk
- ¾ cup sugar, honey or maple syrup
- ½ teaspoon grated cinnamon
- 2 tablespoons extra virgin olive oil
- 2 cups of water
- ½ cup rosewater (optional)

<u>Instructions</u>

1. In a medium pot, put rice and add boiling water. Let the rice boil over low heat until all water evaporates.
2. Add milk until boiled. Stir consistently.
3. Add sugar or honey and rose water (optional) and stir for 3-5 more minutes. Add cinnamon powder on top.
4. Serve warm or cold. Enjoy!

Cooking Tips:

- It is highly recommended to use rosewater in this rice pudding to experience a luxurious taste!
- If you want to have a delicious yellow rice pudding, add ⅓ teaspoon grounded saffron.

Low residue diet-related Tips:

- Always try to consume less sugar. Instead, you can use honey. If you cannot tolerate honey well, you can use maple syrup or stevia.

Nutrition Facts
Servings: 6

Amount per serving	
Calories	**290**
	% Daily Value*
Total Fat 5.7g	7%
Saturated Fat 1.3g	6%
Cholesterol 4mg	1%
Sodium 41mg	2%
Total Carbohydrate 55.3g	20%
Dietary Fiber 0.5g	2%
Total Sugars 27.7g	
Protein 5g	
Vitamin D 42mcg	211%
Calcium 134mg	10%
Iron 2mg	10%
Potassium 239mg	5%

GLUTEN-FREE APPLE PIE

This homemade gluten-free apple pie made with almond flour can satisfy you and your gut!

- Prep Time: 30 minutes
- Cook Time: 55 minutes
- Total Time: 85 minutes
- Serving: 6

Ingredients

- 1¾ cups almond flour, grounded
- ¼ cup tapioca flour+2 tablespoons tapioca flour
- 6 tablespoons extra virgin olive oil
- ½ large egg whisked
- 1 cup rolled oats or gluten-free oats
- 1 cup + ½ tablespoon honey
- 1 teaspoon cinnamon powder
- ½ teaspoon ground ginger
- 4 apples, peeled, cored and sliced
- 1 tablespoon lemon juice
- 1 tablespoon vanilla extract
- Salt, to taste

Instructions

1. In a large bowl, mix almond and tapioca flour rolled oats and olive oil.
2. In a bowl, whisk egg a bit and adds ½ of an egg into the dough. Mix well to form a soft-ball. If the texture is not good, add 1 or 2 teaspoons of the whisked egg to the dough.
3. Put your dough on a parchment paper. Fridge the dough for an hour (Recommended keeping it in a fridge overnight).
4. Remove from the fridge. With a rolling pin, make a 10-12 inch disk. Then, gently move your dough disk

to the pie plate. Return into its shape again if any part falls apart or breaks.
5. Crimp the edges with your fingertips. Make small holes in all parts of your dough.
6. In a large bowl, mix thinly sliced apples with lemon juice, vanilla extract, sugar or honey, ginger, and salt.
7. Cover your crust with the mix altogether.
8. Preheat oven to 400 °F.
9. Cover crust edges with a pie shield to avoid burning fast.
10. Bake for 15-20 minutes. Reduce heat to 350°F and let it bake for 40 minutes.
11. Remove from the oven. Cool down. Slice it and serve.

Cooking Tips:

- Cover the pie with aluminum foil if you see the toppings are getting brown so fast.

Low residue diet-related Tips:

- If you cannot tolerate honey well, you can use maple syrup or stevia.

Nutrition Facts
Servings: 6

Amount per serving	
Calories	**380**
	% Daily Value*
Total Fat 23.4g	30%
Saturated Fat 2.8g	14%
Cholesterol 14mg	5%
Sodium 18mg	1%
Total Carbohydrate 40.5g	15%
Dietary Fiber 6.1g	22%
Total Sugars 16.5g	
Protein 5.3g	
Vitamin D 1mcg	6%
Calcium 43mg	3%
Iron 2mg	10%
Potassium 298mg	6%

PUMPKIN PIE

Enjoy cooking a traditional pumpkin pie recipe for IBD patients!

- Prep Time: 15 minutes
- Cook Time: 55 minutes
- Total Time: 70 minutes
- Serving: 4-6

Ingredients

- 2 cups pumpkin, peeled
- 1 ready pie crust, gluten-free (9-inch)
- 2 organic, free-range eggs
- 1.5 cups condensed milk or lactose-free condensed milk
- ½ teaspoon freshly grated ginger
- ½ teaspoon cinnamon powder
- ½ teaspoon salt

Instructions

1. Preheat oven to 400°F.
2. Blend the pumpkin with all other ingredients in a blender or whisk all ingredients in a large bowl.
3. Pour the mix in a ready crust and bake for 15 minutes.
4. Reduce heat to 350 °F and let it bake for 35-40 minutes. You can insert a fork into it. The fork has to come out very clean, showing that it perfectly cooked.
5. Serve and enjoy!

Cooking Tips:

- Cover the pie with aluminum foil if you see the toppings are getting brown so fast.

Low residue diet-related Tips:

- Make sure you can tolerate condensed milk. If you cannot, use lactose-free cow milk or almond milk instead.

Nutrition Facts	
Servings: 6	
Amount per serving	
Calories	**403**
	% Daily Value*
Total Fat 15.3g	20%
Saturated Fat 5.8g	29%
Cholesterol 81mg	27%
Sodium 258mg	11%
Total Carbohydrate 58.9g	21%
Dietary Fiber 2.6g	9%
Total Sugars 45.3g	
Protein 9.7g	
Vitamin D 5mcg	26%
Calcium 251mg	19%
Iron 2mg	11%
Potassium 497mg	11%

Fruit Dessert

A fresh cold fruit mix as a healthy dessert choice for IBD patients.

- Prep Time: 20 minutes
- Total Time: 20 minutes
- Serving: 4

Ingredients

- 2 cups cantaloupe, cubed
- 1 tablespoon maple syrup
- 3 tablespoons lime juice
- 1 cup papaya, cubed
- 2 cups honeydew melon, cubed

Instructions

1. In a large bowl, mix all ingredients.

2. Serve cold. Enjoy!

Cooking Tips:

- You can change the fruits in your fruit dessert as you wish, but make sure you can tolerate those fruits and always peel them off.
- You can mix your fruits with plain yogurt or lactose-free plain yogurt, as well.

Low residue diet-related Tips:

- Peel and poach fruits such as apple, pear, or peach if you want to add them into your fruit dessert.

Nutrition Facts
Servings: 4

Amount per serving	
Calories	132
	% Daily Value*
Total Fat 0.5g	1%
Saturated Fat 0.1g	1%
Cholesterol 0mg	0%
Sodium 33mg	1%
Total Carbohydrate 34g	12%
Dietary Fiber 3.3g	12%
Total Sugars 27.3g	
Protein 1.8g	
Vitamin D 0mcg	0%
Calcium 36mg	3%
Iron 1mg	4%
Potassium 594mg	13%

Avocado Pear Popsicle

Homemade popsicles are great desserts for people with IBD. It is very easy to make popsicles at home. You need to try this recipe as an example:

- Prep Time: 10 minutes
- Freeze Time: 90 minutes
- Total Time: 100 minutes
- Serving: 4

Ingredients

- 2 avocados, peeled
- 2 pears, peeled and cored

Instructions

1. Blend well pears and avocados in a blender or food processor.
2. Fill up your Popsicle cups. Insert popsicle sticks and freeze.
3. Run the outside of the cup under hot water to remove the popsicles when you want to eat it.

Cooking Tips:

- You can change the fruit(s) in your popsicle as you wish, but make sure you can tolerate those fruits and always peel them off.

Low residue diet-related Tips:

- Peel and poach fruits such as apple, pear, or peach if you want to make a Popsicle from them.

Nutrition Facts	
Servings: 4	
Amount per serving	
Calories	**245**
	% Daily Value*
Total Fat 19.7g	25%
Saturated Fat 4.1g	21%
Cholesterol 0mg	0%
Sodium 7mg	0%
Total Carbohydrate 19.2g	7%
Dietary Fiber 8.9g	32%
Total Sugars 7.3g	
Protein 2.2g	
Vitamin D 0mcg	0%
Calcium 18mg	1%
Iron 1mg	4%
Potassium 568mg	12%

Lemon Sorbet

Try a Paleo-kind refreshing sorbet with great combinations of lemon juice and honey.

- Prep Time: 10 minutes
- Make Time: 120 minutes
- Total Time: 130 minutes
- Serving: 4

Ingredients

- 1 cup fresh lemon juice
- 2 tablespoons lemon zest
- 2 cups of water
- ½ cup honey or maple syrup
- 1 cup light cream
- ¼ teaspoon vanilla extract

Instructions

1. In a medium pot, mix your honey (or maple syrup), lemon zest, and water until the honey dissolves and gets warm.
2. Add lemon juice or squeeze a lemon to the pot. Stir a bit.
3. Pour your sorbet mixture into a metal pan or pot or an ice cream maker.
4. Freeze for 2 hours. Scrape the sorbet with a spoon or fork every 15 minutes.
5. Enjoy!

Cooking Tips:

- You can change the fruit(s) in your sorbet as you wish, but make sure you can tolerate those fruits and always peel them off. Some fruits need to be cooked before making the sorbet.

Low residue diet-related Tips:

- Peel and poach fruits such as apple, pear, or peach if you want to make a sorbet from them.
- Make sure you can tolerate light cream. Instead, you can use almond milk. Be aware that it may need more freezing time if you use almond milk.

Nutrition Facts
Servings: 4

Amount per serving	
Calories	**234**
	% Daily Value*
Total Fat 9.8g	13%
Saturated Fat 6.3g	31%
Cholesterol 33mg	11%
Sodium 24mg	1%
Total Carbohydrate 37.7g	14%
Dietary Fiber 0.5g	2%
Total Sugars 36.3g	
Protein 1.3g	
Vitamin D 0mcg	0%
Calcium 29mg	2%
Iron 0mg	1%
Potassium 136mg	3%

Mango Ice Cream

This dairy-free mango ice cream is very easy to make. It is healthy and a tasty dessert choice for IBD patients.

- Prep Time: 15 minutes
- Cook Time: 30 minutes
- Total Time: 45 minutes
- Serving: 6

Ingredients

- 1¾ cup almond milk
- 2 mangos, peeled

- ¼ cup honey or maple syrup
- ½ teaspoon vanilla extract

Instructions

1. Perfectly chill your almond milk in a fridge before you make this ice cream.
2. Blend milk, mango, maple syrup, and vanilla extract in a blender until perfectly smooth.
3. Pour your sorbet mixture into a metal container, pot, or an ice cream maker. If you use an ice cream maker, it takes about 30 minutes, but if you use a metal container, you may need to freeze it for 90-120 minutes.
4. Serve cold and enjoy it!

Cooking Tips:

- You can change the fruits in your ice cream as you desire, but make sure you can tolerate those fruits and always peel them off. Some fruits need to be cooked before making ice cream.

Low residue diet-related Tips:

- Peel and poach fruits such as apple, pear, or peach if you want to make a sorbet from them.

Nutrition Facts	
Servings: 6	
Amount per serving	
Calories	**272**
	% Daily Value*
Total Fat 17.1g	22%
Saturated Fat 14.9g	75%
Cholesterol 0mg	0%
Sodium 12mg	1%
Total Carbohydrate 32.3g	12%
Dietary Fiber 3.4g	12%
Total Sugars 29.3g	
Protein 2.6g	
Vitamin D 0mcg	0%
Calcium 24mg	2%
Iron 1mg	8%
Potassium 380mg	8%

SWEET POTATO PIE

If you want to make a pie with potato as a dessert, you can follow the recipe of sweet potato pie.

- Prep Time: 30 minutes
- Cook Time: 50 minutes
- Total Time: 80 minutes
- Serving: 4-6

Ingredients

- 2 medium sweet potatoes, peeled and cubed
- ¾ cup condensed milk or lactose-free condensed milk
- 1 deep-dish pie shell, uncooked (or gluten-free pastry shell)
- 2 tablespoons extra virgin olive oil
- ½ cup sugar or 1 tablespoon honey
- 2 large organic, free-range eggs
- 1 teaspoon vanilla extract
- ½ teaspoon cinnamon powder
- ½ teaspoon ground nutmeg
- ¼ teaspoon salt

Instructions

1. In a large pot, boil sweet potatoes by boiling water over medium heat.
2. Drain and mash potatoes by fork or blender.
3. Preheat oven to 400°F.
4. Mix mashed sweet potatoes with extra virgin olive oil, sugar, eggs, cinnamon, vanilla, nutmeg, and salt perfectly in a large bowl.
5. Pour the mix into a ready pie shell. Bake it for 20 minutes. Then, reduce heat around 350 °F and bake for 30-35 more minutes.
6. Serve warm or cold. Enjoy!

Cooking Tips:

- Cover the pie shell with aluminum foil if you see the toppings are getting brown so fast.

Low residue diet-related Tips:

- Make sure you can tolerate nutmeg. If you cannot, remove it from the ingredients.

Nutrition Facts

Servings: 6

Amount per serving	
Calories	**392**
	% Daily Value*
Total Fat 16.6g	21%
Saturated Fat 3.4g	17%
Cholesterol 75mg	25%
Sodium 74mg	3%
Total Carbohydrate 44.8g	16%
Dietary Fiber 1.1g	4%
Total Sugars 37.9g	
Protein 6.5g	
Vitamin D 6mcg	29%
Calcium 122mg	9%
Iron 1mg	3%
Potassium 370mg	8%

WHITE PANNA COTTA

A dairy-free, easy to make panna cotta for IBD patients that comes with a lovely creamy taste of almond milk.

- Prep Time: 10 minutes
- Chill time: 120 minutes
- Total Time: 130 minutes
- Serving: 4

Ingredients

- 1¾ cup almond milk
- ⅓ cup maple syrup or honey
- 2 teaspoons gelatin, grass-fed
- 1 teaspoon vanilla extract

Instructions

1. In a medium pan, heat almond milk and add gelatin. Stir until gelatin powder melts.
2. Add vanilla. Stir and let the mix get warmer for 3-5 minutes over medium heat until gelatin fully dissolved. Be aware that you should not boil the milk.
3. Remove from pan and add maple syrup or honey. Stir well.
4. Fill some small cups with the mixture and fridge it for 3-4 hours.
5. To remove Panna Cotta easily, put small cups in a hot water bowl for 2 minutes. Then, you can flip Panna Cottas on your dessert plates. Enjoy!

Cooking Tips:

- For having a fruity Panna Cotta, you can add poached and peeled fruit cubes in your mixture, as well.

- Alternatively, you can garnish your panna cotta with fruits you can tolerate.

Low residue diet-related Tips:

Nutrition Facts	
Servings: 4	
Amount per serving	
Calories	**325**
	% Daily Value*
Total Fat 25.1g	32%
Saturated Fat 22.2g	111%
Cholesterol 0mg	0%
Sodium 25mg	1%
Total Carbohydrate 23.6g	9%
Dietary Fiber 2.3g	8%
Total Sugars 19.3g	
Protein 5.4g	
Vitamin D 0mcg	0%
Calcium 36mg	3%
Iron 2mg	12%
Potassium 332mg	7%

COCKTAILS AND SHAKES

BANANA MILKSHAKE

Enjoy tasting a traditional milkshake with banana.

- Prep Time: 5 minutes
- Serving: 1

Ingredients

- 1 banana
- 1 cup unsweetened almond or lactose-free milk
- ½ teaspoon stevia or two tablespoons honey or maple syrup

Instructions

- Blend all the above ingredients until smooth. Pour into a large glass. Enjoy!

Cooking Tips:

- You can use plain lactose-free yogurt or banana lactose-free yogurt instead of milk.
- Use agave syrup if you cannot tolerate maple syrup or honey.

Low residue diet-related Tips:

- Use honey only if you can tolerate it.

Nutrition Facts	
Servings: 1	
Amount per serving	
Calories	**145**
	% Daily Value*
Total Fat 3.9g	5%
Saturated Fat 0.4g	2%
Cholesterol 0mg	0%
Sodium 181mg	8%
Total Carbohydrate 29g	11%
Dietary Fiber 4.1g	15%
Total Sugars 14.4g	
Protein 2.3g	
Vitamin D 1mcg	7%
Calcium 306mg	24%
Iron 1mg	6%
Potassium 612mg	13%

Cooler Drink

Enjoy tasting a great drink that makes you really cool!

- Prep Time: 5 minutes
- Serving: 1

Ingredients

- 2 cucumbers, peeled
- 10 mint leaves
- 1 cup lemon juice
- 1 cup of water
- Ice cubes

Instructions

- Blend all ingredients in a blender and then blend until smooth. Pour into a large glass. Enjoy!

Cooking Tips:

- You can add one teaspoon of freshly grated ginger to the drink as well.

Nutrition Facts	
Servings: 1	
Amount per serving	
Calories	**193**
	% Daily Value*
Total Fat 3.3g	4%
Saturated Fat 2.4g	12%
Cholesterol 0mg	0%
Sodium 91mg	4%
Total Carbohydrate 35.4g	13%
Dietary Fiber 10.8g	39%
Total Sugars 15.2g	
Protein 9.2g	
Vitamin D 0mcg	0%
Calcium 312mg	24%
Iron 14mg	76%
Potassium 1646mg	35%

Mango-Banana Smoothie

A great smoothie with mango and banana!

- Prep Time: 5 minutes
- Serving: 1-2

Ingredients

- 1 mango, diced
- 1 banana, diced
- 1 cup lactose-free milk or almond milk
- ½ teaspoon stevia (or honey or maple syrup)

Instructions

- Blend all ingredients in a blender and then blend until smooth. Pour into a large glass. Enjoy!

Cooking Tips:

- You can use plain lactose-free yogurt or banana lactose-free yogurt instead of milk for having a thick texture.
- Use agave syrup if you cannot tolerate maple syrup or honey.

Low residue diet-related Tips:

- Use honey only if you can tolerate it.
- If you cannot tolerate mango, use papaya instead.

Nutrition Facts	
Servings: 2	
Amount per serving	
Calories	**218**
	% Daily Value*
Total Fat 3.4g	4%
Saturated Fat 1.7g	9%
Cholesterol 11mg	4%
Sodium 62mg	3%
Total Carbohydrate 44.7g	16%
Dietary Fiber 4.2g	15%
Total Sugars 30.2g	
Protein 6.3g	
Vitamin D 50mcg	250%
Calcium 171mg	13%
Iron 0mg	2%
Potassium 703mg	15%

GINGER COOL DRINK

A great healthy drink for IBD patients.

- Prep Time: 5 minutes
- Serving: 1

Ingredients

- 5 tablespoons applesauce

- 1 cup of water
- 1 cup of cooked pear or 1 can of pear compote
- 1 small piece of ginger or 2 teaspoons ginger powder

Instructions

- Blend all ingredients in a blender and then blend until smooth. Pour into a large glass. Enjoy!

Cooking Tips:

- You can use lactose-free milk or almond milk instead of water to make a great smoothie.
- You can add honey (if you can tolerate) or ½ tablespoon of stevia for sweetness.

Nutrition Facts	
Servings: 1	
Amount per serving	
Calories	138
	% Daily Value*
Total Fat 0.5g	1%
Saturated Fat 0.1g	0%
Cholesterol 0mg	0%
Sodium 5mg	0%
Total Carbohydrate 35.7g	13%
Dietary Fiber 6.4g	23%
Total Sugars 23.5g	
Protein 1g	
Vitamin D 0mcg	0%
Calcium 21mg	2%
Iron 1mg	4%
Potassium 292mg	6%

Avocado Smoothie

A great healthy drink for IBD patients with healthy fats. If you like, you can add protein powder in the smoothie.

- Prep Time: 5 minutes
- Serving: 1-2

Ingredients

- 1 avocado
- 1 banana
- 1 cup lactose-free milk or unsweetened almond milk
- 2 tablespoons maple syrup or 1 teaspoon stevia

Instructions

- Blend all ingredients in a blender and then blend until smooth. Pour into a large glass. Enjoy!

Cooking Tips:

- Use can use honey (if you can tolerate) instead of maple syrup.

Nutrition Facts
Servings: 2

Amount per serving	
Calories	**375**
	% Daily Value*
Total Fat 22.3g	29%
Saturated Fat 5.7g	29%
Cholesterol 10mg	3%
Sodium 71mg	3%
Total Carbohydrate 42g	15%
Dietary Fiber 8.3g	30%
Total Sugars 25.6g	
Protein 6.6g	
Vitamin D 0mcg	0%
Calcium 178mg	14%
Iron 1mg	6%
Potassium 730mg	16%

Banana-Cinnamon Smoothie

A classical thick smoothie to enjoy!

- Prep Time: 5 minutes
- Serving: 1

Ingredients

- 1 banana
- 1 cup vanilla yogurt or lactose-free yogurt

- 2 teaspoons maple syrup or ½ teaspoon stevia
- 1 teaspoon cinnamon
- ⅓ cup of ice

Instructions

- Blend all ingredients in a blender and then blend until smooth. Pour into a large glass. Enjoy!

Cooking Tips:

- Use can use honey (if you can tolerate) instead of maple syrup.
- Plain yogurt can also be used instead of vanilla yogurt.

Nutrition Facts
Servings: 1

Amount per serving	
Calories	**320**
	% Daily Value*
Total Fat 3.5g	4%
Saturated Fat 2.6g	13%
Cholesterol 15mg	5%
Sodium 174mg	8%
Total Carbohydrate 55g	20%
Dietary Fiber 4.3g	15%
Total Sugars 39.7g	
Protein 15.3g	
Vitamin D 0mcg	0%
Calcium 486mg	37%
Iron 1mg	5%
Potassium 1033mg	22%

Peach-Mango-Banana Smoothie

A fabulous smoothie with three different fruits to enjoy!

- Prep Time: 5 minutes
- Serving: 1-2

Ingredients

- ½ mango, diced

- ½ banana, diced
- 1 peach, diced and skin-removed
- 1 cup plain yogurt or lactose-free yogurt
- ½ cup of ice
- 1 teaspoon stevia (or honey or maple syrup)

Instructions

- Blend all ingredients in a blender and then blend until smooth. Pour into a large glass. Enjoy!

Cooking Tips:

- You can use two tablespoons of agave syrup, honey, or sugar instead of stevia if you can tolerate it.

Low residue diet-related Tips:

- Use honey only if you can tolerate it.
- If you cannot tolerate mango, use papaya instead.

Nutrition Facts	
Servings: 1	
Amount per serving	
Calories	387
	% Daily Value*
Total Fat 4.2g	5%
Saturated Fat 2.7g	13%
Cholesterol 15mg	5%
Sodium 174mg	8%
Total Carbohydrate 69.9g	25%
Dietary Fiber 6.5g	23%
Total Sugars 61.4g	
Protein 17.4g	
Vitamin D 0mcg	0%
Calcium 470mg	36%
Iron 1mg	5%
Potassium 1352mg	29%

PEACH-GINGER SMOOTHIE

A ginger-based smoothie with a fantastic taste!

- Prep Time: 5 minutes

- Serving: 1

Ingredients

- 1 peach, diced and skin-removed
- 1 cup lactose-free milk or unsweetened almond milk
- 1 tablespoon fresh grated ginger
- 1 teaspoon stevia (or one tablespoon honey or maple syrup)

Instructions

- Blend all ingredients in a blender and then blend until smooth. Pour into a large glass. Enjoy!

Cooking Tips:

- You can use two tablespoons of agave syrup, honey, or sugar instead of stevia if you can tolerate it.

Low residue diet-related Tips:

- Use honey only if you can tolerate it.

Nutrition Facts	
Servings: 1	
Amount per serving	
Calories	**208**
	% Daily Value*
Total Fat 5.7g	7%
Saturated Fat 3.1g	16%
Cholesterol 20mg	7%
Sodium 127mg	6%
Total Carbohydrate 30.8g	11%
Dietary Fiber 3g	11%
Total Sugars 26.2g	
Protein 9.9g	
Vitamin D 0mcg	0%
Calcium 306mg	24%
Iron 1mg	5%
Potassium 358mg	8%

POMEGRANATE-ANGELICA SMOOTHIE

Enjoy a healthy smoothie with a fantastic sour taste!

- Prep Time: 5 minutes
- Serving: 1-2

Ingredients

- 1 cup pomegranate juice
- ½ cup plain yogurt or lactose-free yogurt
- 1 tablespoon Angelica root powder (optional)
- 1 teaspoon salt

Instructions

- Blend all ingredients in a blender and then blend until smooth. Pour into a large glass. Enjoy!

Cooking Tips:

- You can use one tablespoon of honey or maple syrup for giving sweetness to the smoothie if you can tolerate it.

Low residue diet-related Tips:

- Use honey only if you can tolerate it.
- Make sure you are not eating pomegranate seeds.

Nutrition Facts	
Servings: 1	
Amount per serving	
Calories	**237**
	% Daily Value*
Total Fat 1.5g	2%
Saturated Fat 1.2g	6%
Cholesterol 7mg	2%
Sodium 2421mg	105%
Total Carbohydrate 45.6g	17%
Dietary Fiber 0g	0%
Total Sugars 40.6g	
Protein 7g	
Vitamin D 0mcg	0%
Calcium 246mg	19%
Iron 0mg	1%
Potassium 887mg	19%

APPLE-GINGER SMOOTHIE

A ginger-based smoothie with a fantastic taste!

- Prep Time: 5 minutes
- Serving: 1-2

Ingredients

- 1 apple, diced and skin-removed
- 1 cup lactose-free milk or unsweetened almond milk
- 3 tablespoons lime juice
- 1 tablespoon fresh grated ginger
- 1 tablespoon honey

Instructions

- Blend all ingredients in a blender and then blend until smooth. Pour into a large glass. Enjoy!

Cooking Tips:

- You can use one tablespoon of maple syrup, or one teaspoon of stevia instead of honey.

Low residue diet-related Tips:

- Use honey only if you can tolerate it.

Nutrition Facts	
Servings: 1	
Amount per serving	
Calories	**345**
	% Daily Value*
Total Fat 5.8g	7%
Saturated Fat 3.1g	16%
Cholesterol 20mg	7%
Sodium 131mg	6%
Total Carbohydrate 70.5g	26%
Dietary Fiber 6.4g	23%
Total Sugars 53.7g	
Protein 9.4g	
Vitamin D 0mcg	0%
Calcium 318mg	24%
Iron 2mg	10%
Potassium 399mg	8%

Bloody Red Drink!

Enjoy a healthy drink with an amazing sour taste!

- Prep Time: 5 minutes
- Serving: 1-2

Ingredients

- 1 cup pomegranate juice
- ½ beet juice
- ½ tablespoon Angelica powder
- 1 teaspoon salt
- 1 tablespoon honey (or maple syrup), to taste

Instructions

- Blend all the ingredients in a blender until smooth. Pour into a large glass. Enjoy!

Cooking Tips:

- You can use one teaspoon of stevia instead of honey or maple syrup.

Low residue diet-related Tips:

- If you are experiencing a flare-up, remove the beet from the recipe.
- Use honey only if you can tolerate it.

Nutrition Facts	
Servings: 1	
Amount per serving	
Calories	267
	% Daily Value*
Total Fat 0g	0%
Saturated Fat 0g	0%
Cholesterol 0mg	0%
Sodium 2384mg	104%
Total Carbohydrate 66.3g	24%
Dietary Fiber 0g	0%
Total Sugars 60.3g	
Protein 1.6g	
Vitamin D 0mcg	0%
Calcium 23mg	2%
Iron 0mg	1%
Potassium 611mg	13%

Papaya-Mango Smoothie

Enjoy a great combination of papaya and mango in a refreshing smoothie!

- Prep Time: 5-7 minutes
- Serving: 2

Ingredients

- 1 cup mango, diced
- 1 cup papaya chunks
- 1 cup almond or lactose-free milk
- 1 tablespoon honey or maple syrup

Instructions

- Blend all ingredients in a blender and then blend until smooth. Pour into a large glass. Enjoy!

Cooking Tips:

- You can use one teaspoon of stevia instead of honey or maple syrup.

Low residue diet-related Tips:

- Use honey only if you can tolerate it.
- If mango irritates your gut, use papaya instead.

Nutrition Facts	
Servings: 2	
Amount per serving	
Calories	**398**
	% Daily Value*
Total Fat 29g	37%
Saturated Fat 25.5g	127%
Cholesterol 0mg	0%
Sodium 20mg	1%
Total Carbohydrate 38.5g	14%
Dietary Fiber 5.1g	18%
Total Sugars 32g	
Protein 3.9g	
Vitamin D 0mcg	0%
Calcium 39mg	3%
Iron 2mg	13%
Potassium 550mg	12%

Cantaloupe Smoothie

Enjoy a great smoothie with cantaloupe!

- Prep Time: 5 minutes
- Serving: 1-2

Ingredients

- 1 cup cantaloupe, diced
- ½ cup vanilla yogurt or lactose-free yogurt
- ½ cup of orange juice
- 1 tablespoon honey (or maple syrup), to taste
- 2 ice cubes

Instructions

- Blend all ingredients in a blender and then blend until smooth. Pour into a large glass. Enjoy!

Cooking Tips:

- You can use 1 teaspoon of stevia instead of honey or maple syrup.

Low residue diet-related Tips:

- Use honey only if you can tolerate it.
- If orange juice irritates your gut, simply remove it from the recipe.

Nutrition Facts	
Servings: 1	
Amount per serving	
Calories	260
	% Daily Value*
Total Fat 2.1g	3%
Saturated Fat 1.4g	7%
Cholesterol 7mg	2%
Sodium 113mg	5%
Total Carbohydrate 51.6g	19%
Dietary Fiber 1.7g	6%
Total Sugars 48.5g	
Protein 9.2g	
Vitamin D 0mcg	0%
Calcium 241mg	19%
Iron 2mg	11%
Potassium 962mg	20%

Cantaloupe-Mix Smoothie

Enjoy a great mix of cantaloupe with mango, lemon, and orange!

- Prep Time: 5-10 minutes
- Serving: 2

Ingredients

- 1 cup cantaloupe, diced
- ½ cup mango, diced

- ½ cup almond milk or lactose-free cow milk
- ½ cup of orange juice
- 2 tablespoons lemon
- 1 tablespoon honey (or maple syrup), to taste
- 2 ice cubes

Instructions

- Blend the ingredients in a blender until smooth. Pour into a large glass. Enjoy!

Cooking Tips:

- You can use one teaspoon of stevia instead of honey or maple syrup.

Low residue diet-related Tips:

- Use honey only if you can tolerate it.
- If orange juice irritates your gut, remove it from the recipe.
- If you cannot tolerate mango, use papaya instead.

Nutrition Facts
Servings: 2

Amount per serving	
Calories	**253**
	% Daily Value*
Total Fat 14.8g	19%
Saturated Fat 12.8g	64%
Cholesterol 0mg	0%
Sodium 23mg	1%
Total Carbohydrate 32.2g	12%
Dietary Fiber 3.2g	11%
Total Sugars 27.9g	
Protein 3g	
Vitamin D 0mcg	0%
Calcium 26mg	2%
Iron 2mg	12%
Potassium 583mg	12%

Applesauce-Avocado Smoothie

Have you tried the taste of applesauce with avocado? Try this smoothie cold!

- Prep Time: 5-7 minutes
- Serving: 1

Ingredients

- 1 cup unsweetened almond or lactose-free milk
- ½ avocado
- ½ cup applesauce
- ¼ teaspoon ground cinnamon
- ½ cup ice

Instructions

- Blend all ingredients in a blender. Blend the mix until smooth. Pour into a large glass. Enjoy!

Cooking Tips:

- You can use ½ teaspoon of stevia or 1 tablespoon of honey for sweetness.

Nutrition Facts
Servings: 1

Amount per serving	
Calories	**299**
	% Daily Value*
Total Fat 23.2g	30%
Saturated Fat 4.4g	22%
Cholesterol 0mg	0%
Sodium 189mg	8%
Total Carbohydrate 24.9g	9%
Dietary Fiber 9.5g	34%
Total Sugars 12.8g	
Protein 3.1g	
Vitamin D 1mcg	7%
Calcium 322mg	25%
Iron 2mg	8%
Potassium 771mg	16%

PINA COLADA SMOOTHIE

A classical gluten-free Mexican smoothie for your parties!

- Prep Time: 5 minutes
- Serving: 1

Ingredients

- 1 cup papaya chunks
- ½ cup unsweetened almond milk or lactose-free milk
- 1 banana
- ½ teaspoon vanilla extract, to taste
- 1 tablespoon honey, maple syrup or one teaspoon stevia (optional)

Instructions

- Blend all ingredients in a blender and then blend until smooth and creamy. Pour into a large glass. Enjoy!

Cooking Tips:

- For sweetness, you can add stevia, honey, or maple syrup as instructed.

Low residue diet-related Tips:

- Use honey only if you can tolerate it.

Nutrition Facts	
Servings: 1	
Amount per serving	
Calories	**348**
	% Daily Value*
Total Fat 9g	12%
Saturated Fat 6.2g	31%
Cholesterol 0mg	0%
Sodium 98mg	4%
Total Carbohydrate 70.2g	26%
Dietary Fiber 7.7g	28%
Total Sugars 49.4g	
Protein 3.4g	
Vitamin D 1mcg	3%
Calcium 179mg	14%
Iron 4mg	22%
Potassium 783mg	17%

SNACKS

DICED FRUITS

You can dice fresh fruits you can tolerate and use them between your daily main meals. Papaya, honeydew melon, cantaloupe, and banana are some of the best fruits for IBD patients.

PLAIN YOGURT WITH POACHED FRUITS

Another great snack is mixing plain/vanilla yogurt or lactose-free plain or vanilla yogurt with fruits you can tolerate or peeled and poached fruits. As explained, papaya, honeydew melon, cantaloupe, and banana are some of the best fruits for IBD patients. The following recipe shows how to poach fruits like apple and peach to make a delicious homemade compote.

POACHED FRUIT COMPOTE

It is a great choice that can be consumed by IBD patients.

- Prep Time: 10 minutes
- Cook Time: 40 Minutes

- Total Time: 50 minutes
- Serving: 6

Ingredients

- 4 peaches, skin removed and thinly sliced
- 1 lb apple, pitted and skin removed
- 1 teaspoon cinnamon powder
- 1 cup honey or maple syrup
- 1 teaspoon vanilla extract

Instructions

1. In a large pot, cook fruits in boiling water over medium heat until softened.
2. In a large bowl, mix well all ingredients (except fruits) together.
3. Pour the syrup over fruits and let the compote be thickened.
4. Pour compote into a jar. Serve hot or cold. Enjoy!

Cooking Tips:

- You can poach fruits with the skin and remove the skin after poaching and before adding syrup to it.
- If you can tolerate sugar and for better sweetness, you can use ½ cup of cane sugar.
- You can poach other fruits such as pear with the same instructions.

Low residue diet-related Tips:

- Make sure you wash fruits thoroughly after peeling them off.
- Some IBD patients cannot tolerate peach. Always make and consume poached fruits you can tolerate.

Nutrition Facts	
Servings: 6	
Amount per serving	
Calories	**232**
	% Daily Value*
Total Fat 0.3g	0%
Saturated Fat 0g	0%
Cholesterol 0mg	0%
Sodium 3mg	0%
Total Carbohydrate 61.1g	22%
Dietary Fiber 2.5g	9%
Total Sugars 59.7g	
Protein 1.2g	
Vitamin D 0mcg	0%
Calcium 4mg	0%
Iron 1mg	4%
Potassium 260mg	6%

APPLESAUCE

Applesauce is a fantastic option for people who are following the low residue diet. You can purchase applesauce from different stores. It is recommended to use organic applesauce, or you can make it at home:

HOMEMADE APPLESAUCE

- Prep Time: 10 minutes
- Cook Time: 30 Minutes
- Total Time: 40 minutes
- Serving: 4

Ingredients

- 6 organic apples, peeled, cored and cubed
- ½ cup boiling water
- ½ teaspoon cinnamon powder
- ¼ cup sugar or four tablespoons honey
- 2 tablespoons fresh lemon juice
- ¼ teaspoon salt

Instructions

1. In a large pot, cook apples with boiling water, lemon juice, cinnamon, sugar or honey, and salt over medium-low heat until softened. Remove from heat.
2. You can mash all ingredients by using a fork or blend with a blender or a food processor.
3. Pour applesauce into a suitable container or jar. Serve warm or cold. Enjoy!

Cooking Tips:

- Pink lady apples are preferable for making delicious applesauce.

Low residue diet-related Tips:

- Make sure you wash apples thoroughly after peeling them off.
- If you cannot tolerate sugar or honey well, you may add one tablespoon of Stevia instead.

Nutrition Facts
Servings: 4

Amount per serving
Calories   **223**

	% Daily Value*
Total Fat 0.7g	1%
Saturated Fat 0.1g	0%
Cholesterol 0mg	0%
Sodium 5mg	0%
Total Carbohydrate 58.9g	21%
Dietary Fiber 8.1g	29%
Total Sugars 47.5g	
Protein 1g	
Vitamin D 0mcg	0%
Calcium 3mg	0%
Iron 2mg	8%
Potassium 368mg	8%

AVOCADO DIP

A modified avocado dip recipe is a great snack candidate for IBD patients.

- Prep Time: 5 minutes
- Cook Time: 0 minutes
- Total Time: 5 minutes
- Serving: 4-6

Ingredients

- 6 avocados, peeled
- ½ tablespoon extra virgin olive oil
- ¼ cup chopped fresh cilantro
- 2 tablespoons fresh lime juice
- 1 teaspoon fresh lemon juice
- ½ teaspoon salt

Instructions

1. In a large bowl, mash avocados with a fork.
2. Add extra virgin olive oil and other ingredients into it.
3. Enjoy!

Cooking Tips:

- You can serve guacamole with tacos if you can tolerate it.
- If you can tolerate a few tomatoes and onions, cube them and then add them into your guacamole.

Low residue diet-related Tips:

- Do not use fresh cilantro if you are experiencing a severe flare-up. Do not take taco chips, as well.

Nutrition Facts	
Servings: 6	
Amount per serving	
Calories	**422**
	% Daily Value*
Total Fat 40.4g	52%
Saturated Fat 8.4g	42%
Cholesterol 0mg	0%
Sodium 207mg	9%
Total Carbohydrate 18g	7%
Dietary Fiber 13.5g	48%
Total Sugars 1.2g	
Protein 3.9g	
Vitamin D 0mcg	0%
Calcium 26mg	2%
Iron 1mg	7%
Potassium 988mg	21%

Homemade Hummus

A healthy and tasty middle-eastern snack. An excellent option for vegetarians and IBD patients during the remission period.

- Prep Time: 5 minutes
- Cook Time: 60 minutes
- Total Time: 65 minutes
- Serving: 4

Ingredients

- ¼ lb dried chickpeas (soaked in water for one night)
- 1½ tablespoon tahini
- 1 tablespoon lemon juice
- 2 tablespoons extra virgin olive oil, divided
- ¼ teaspoon cumin
- ½ teaspoon salt
- 1 tablespoon water
- 1 teaspoon baking soda (optional)
- 1 teaspoon paprika powder (optional)

Instructions

1. First, IBD patients need to soak the chickpeas overnight in water and optionally add baking soda to the water.
2. Cook your chickpeas in a large pot with water, over medium heat for about one hour. Check if chickpeas cooked well by crushing one of them with a fork in your hand.
3. When chickpeas cooked, drain them and put them in a blender.
4. Add 1 tablespoon of extra virgin olive oil, lemon juice, tahini, cumin powder, and salt to the blender. Blend until your hummus gets a soft, creamy texture equally.
5. Sprinkle with one tablespoon extra virgin olive oil or paprika powder (optional).
6. Serve immediately or fridge it.

Cooking Tips:

- Hummus is well-matched with white pita bread.
- You can serve hummus, hot or cold.

Low residue diet-related Tips:

- Do not use paprika in hummus if you are experiencing a severe flare-up.
- Eat hummus in moderation when you are in remission. It is better to avoid making Hummus during flares, or make and eat a little bit of it.

Nutrition Facts	
Servings: 4	
Amount per serving	
Calories	**198**
	% Daily Value*
Total Fat 11.8g	15%
Saturated Fat 1.6g	8%
Cholesterol 0mg	0%
Sodium 305mg	13%
Total Carbohydrate 18.5g	7%
Dietary Fiber 5.5g	20%
Total Sugars 3.1g	
Protein 6.5g	
Vitamin D 0mcg	0%
Calcium 56mg	4%
Iron 2mg	13%
Potassium 279mg	6%

TOFU

Tofu is a fantastic snack option for IBD patients. It is based on soy milk and is rich in calcium and Iron, needed for most IBD patients. Here is a sample recipe of a snack with Tofu:

AVOCADO TOFU TOAST

Enjoy a healthy and rich daily snack!

- Prep Time: 10 minutes
- Cook Time: 35 minutes
- Total Time: 45 minutes
- Serving: 4

Ingredients

- 1½ cup firm tofu, pressed and drained
- 1 avocado, cubed
- 1 tablespoon extra virgin olive oil
- Salt and pepper, to taste

Instructions

1. Preheat your oven to 400 °F.

2. Choose a baking sheet, cover it with parchment paper or spray extra virgin olive oil. Cut tofu-like cubes of 1.5 inches and spray extra virgin olive oil on it.
3. Let it bake for 15 minutes until golden brown and crispy. Flip tofu and cook for another 10 minutes. Remove from the oven. Let it rest for 10 minutes.
4. Cube avocado on a plate and add salt and pepper.
5. Mix the tofu with avocado in a bowl. Enjoy!

Cooking Tips:

- You may want to add one tablespoon of lemon juice to create another great taste.

Low residue diet-related Tips:

- Do not use pepper in this toast if you are experiencing a flare-up.

Nutrition Facts
Servings: 4

Amount per serving	
Calories	**199**
	% Daily Value*
Total Fat 17.2g	22%
Saturated Fat 3.4g	17%
Cholesterol 0mg	0%
Sodium 14mg	1%
Total Carbohydrate 5.9g	2%
Dietary Fiber 4.2g	15%
Total Sugars 0.8g	
Protein 8.7g	
Vitamin D 0mcg	0%
Calcium 196mg	15%
Iron 2mg	10%
Potassium 384mg	8%

ALMOND BUTTER SANDWICH

Almond butter is a fantastic source of fiber and magnesium for IBD patients. It is recommended to use smooth almond butter.

- Prep Time: 5 minutes
- Total Time: 5 minutes
- Serving: 1

Ingredients

- 2 slices of white bread or white gluten-free bread
- 1 tablespoon organic smooth almond butter

Instructions

1. Spread one piece of bread with almond butter.
2. Toast and enjoy!

Cooking Tips:

- You can combine the almond butter sandwich with almond milk or lactose-free cow milk perfectly.

Low residue diet-related Tips:

- Remember to use smooth almond butter if you have large intestinal strictures due to the IBD.

Nutrition Facts

Servings: 1

Amount per serving	
Calories	313
	% Daily Value*
Total Fat 17.7g	23%
Saturated Fat 1.9g	9%
Cholesterol 0mg	0%
Sodium 341mg	15%
Total Carbohydrate 32.3g	12%
Dietary Fiber 5.2g	19%
Total Sugars 4.2g	
Protein 8.8g	
Vitamin D 0mcg	0%
Calcium 156mg	12%
Iron 3mg	16%
Potassium 280mg	6%

GLUTEN-FREE MUFFINS

You may eat different types of muffins, but you have to make sure about the ingredients. The muffin should not be made with fruits you cannot tolerate. Moreover, try not to eat muffins that are made with whole wheat flour. If you are gluten-intolerant or suffering from UC, you can make your muffins at home:

- Prep Time: 15 minutes
- Cook Time: 45 minutes
- Total Time: 60 minutes
- Serving: 5-10 (10 Muffins)

Ingredients

- 2 tablespoons extra virgin olive oil or avocado oil
- 2½ cups almond flour, blanched
- 3 large organic free-range eggs
- ¼ cup organic maple syrup
- 2 teaspoons vanilla extract
- ¼ cup banana, mashed
- 1 teaspoon lemon juice
- ¾ teaspoon baking soda
- ¼ teaspoon cinnamon powder
- ½ teaspoon salt

Instructions

1. Preheat your oven to 375 °F.
2. In a large bowl, mix almond flour, cinnamon, baking soda, and salt. Whisk well.
3. In another bowl, add extra virgin olive oil, vanilla extract, eggs, ripe banana, maple syrup, and lemon juice. Whisk well.
4. Mix the two bowls and stir well with a wooden spoon until flour mixed well with other ingredients.

5. Prepare ten muffin cups. Pour them to the top and then bake for 15 minutes.
6. To avoid browning quickly, loosely cover muffins with an aluminum foil. Cook for another 15 minutes.
7. Put a toothpick in a muffin to check if it cooks well or not. If cooked well, the toothpick should not stick to the muffin.
8. Remove from the oven. Let the muffins cool for 15 more minutes. Enjoy!

Cooking Tips:

- You need to use finely grounded skin removed flour.

Low residue diet-related Tips:

Nutrition Facts	
Servings: 10	
Amount per serving	
Calories	**366**
	% Daily Value*
Total Fat 30.7g	39%
Saturated Fat 2.9g	14%
Cholesterol 65mg	22%
Sodium 242mg	11%
Total Carbohydrate 16.1g	6%
Dietary Fiber 5.1g	18%
Total Sugars 7.8g	
Protein 12.8g	
Vitamin D 0mcg	0%
Calcium 132mg	10%
Iron 2mg	11%
Potassium 31mg	1%

CHEESE STICKS

Cheese sticks are excellent sources of calcium. If you are in remission, you may consume cheese sticks as snacks. Remember to choose low fat or fat-free options. If you are lactose-intolerant, you may use lactose-free Swiss, Havarti, or aged cheddar. One cheddar cheese sticks have the following nutrition fact:

Nutrition Facts	
Servings: 1	
Amount per serving	
Calories	**110**
	% Daily Value*
Total Fat 9g	12%
Saturated Fat 5g	25%
Cholesterol 30mg	10%
Sodium 180mg	8%
Total Carbohydrate 0g	0%
Dietary Fiber 0g	0%
Total Sugars 0g	
Protein 7g	
Vitamin D 0mcg	0%
Calcium 200mg	15%
Iron 0mg	0%
Potassium 0mg	0%

Avocado Tuna Toast

A very fast sandwich you can prepare at home.

- Prep Time: 10 minutes
- Cook Time: 0 minutes
- Total Time: 10 minutes
- Serving: 4

Ingredients

- 2 avocados
- 2 tablespoons organic low-fat mayonnaise
- 1 teaspoon cumin powder
- 1 can of tuna in olive oil or water
- ¼ cup apple, chopped and peeled off
- 4 white toasts or any gluten-free bread
- Salt to taste
- Pepper to taste (optional)

Instructions

1. Choose a small bowl. Mix tuna with smashed avocado with mayo, cumin powder, peeled off apple (cut into small pieces), salt, and pepper (optional).

2. Place tuna mix on two toast slices. Cover with other slices.
3. Toast and enjoy!

Cooking Tips:

- You can make this sandwich without mayonnaise sauce, as well.

Low residue diet-related Tips:

- Do not use black pepper, or cumin powder, if you are experiencing a flare-up.

Nutrition Facts	
Servings: 4	
Amount per serving	
Calories	**386**
	% Daily Value*
Total Fat 26.7g	34%
Saturated Fat 5.2g	26%
Cholesterol 17mg	6%
Sodium 268mg	12%
Total Carbohydrate 23.3g	8%
Dietary Fiber 7.7g	27%
Total Sugars 3g	
Protein 15.8g	
Vitamin D 0mcg	0%
Calcium 45mg	3%
Iron 2mg	11%
Potassium 689mg	15%

Rice Crackers

Most rice crackers in the market are gluten-free and tasty snacks for IBD patients. White rice is an excellent carbohydrate for people with IBD.

Gluten-Free Rice Cracker

A great example of making a rice cracker as a snack.

- Prep Time: 10 minutes
- Cook Time: 15 minutes

- Total Time: 25 minutes
- Serving: 6

Ingredients

- 1 cup white rice flour
- 2 tablespoons extra virgin olive oil
- ⅓ cup of water
- ½ tablespoon salt
- 1 teaspoon honey (optional)

Instructions

1. Preheat oven to 350 °F.
2. In a large bowl, mix white rice flour with oil, salt, honey, and water to create a smooth dough.
3. Roll out the dough on a floured surface and make round, thin rice cookies.
4. Make holes throughout rice cookies by using a fork. Spray them with extra virgin olive oil.
5. Bake crackers for about 15 minutes until slightly golden. Enjoy!

Cooking Tips:

- You can make this cracker in a large pan, as well. Just bake them with extra virgin olive oil over low heat until golden both sides.

Low residue diet-related Tips:

- Make sure you are using white rice flour and no other types of rice flours such as brown rice flours.

Nutrition Facts	
Servings: 6	
Amount per serving	
Calories	**190**
	% Daily Value*
Total Fat 5.2g	7%
Saturated Fat 0.7g	3%
Cholesterol 0mg	0%
Sodium 582mg	25%
Total Carbohydrate 32g	12%
Dietary Fiber 1g	4%
Total Sugars 0g	
Protein 2g	
Vitamin D 0mcg	0%
Calcium 1mg	0%
Iron 0mg	0%
Potassium 0mg	0%

GINGER BISCUITS

Ginger is rich in potassium and vitamin B6 with excellent anti-inflammatory properties. Hence, ginger-based snacks are great snack options for IBD patients.

GLUTEN-FREE GINGER BISCUITS

Enjoy making a gluten-free, dairy-free ginger biscuit in your home.

- Prep Time: 15 minutes
- Cook Time: 20 minutes
- Total Time: 35 minutes
- Serving: 4-6

Ingredients

- ¾ cup shortening or half a cup + 1 tablespoon extra virgin olive oil
- 2 cups gluten-free flour or grated almond flour
- 2 tablespoons honey
- 1 organic, free-range egg
- 2 teaspoons baking soda
- ¼ cup molasses

- 1½ teaspoons freshly grated ginger
- 1 teaspoon cinnamon powder
- ½ teaspoon salt

Instructions

1. In a large bowl, mix oil (or shortening), sugar, molasses, and egg.
2. In another large bowl, mix flour, ginger, baking soda, cinnamon, and salt.
3. Slowly combine ingredients of both bowls until making a soft dough.
4. Let the dough rest for 45 minutes.
5. Preheat oven to 375°F.
6. Roll the dough and make 2-inch (5cm) balls. Pour honey on dough balls.
7. Use cookie sheets with parchment paper. Put balls on cooking sheets and bake for 12-15 minutes until seeing cracks and until having a light brown color.
8. Remove from the oven and cool biscuits for five minutes. Enjoy!

Cooking Tips:

- Shortening gives you a better ginger biscuit texture. However, IBD patients may not tolerate it well. Alternatively, use olive oil.
- If you cannot tolerate honey, you can use a little bit of sugar or maple syrup.
- You can substitute ¼ cup of molasses with ¼ cup maple syrup.

Low residue diet-related Tips:

- Do not use molasses if you cannot tolerate it. Instead, use maple syrup.

Nutrition Facts	
Servings: 6	
Amount per serving	
Calories	**367**
	% Daily Value*
Total Fat 4.5g	6%
Saturated Fat 1.1g	5%
Cholesterol 27mg	9%
Sodium 660mg	29%
Total Carbohydrate 77.2g	28%
Dietary Fiber 8.5g	30%
Total Sugars 15.3g	
Protein 5.6g	
Vitamin D 3mcg	13%
Calcium 34mg	3%
Iron 1mg	6%
Potassium 236mg	5%

ZUCCHINI CHIPS

Zucchini chips are a healthy, low-calorie snack for IBD patients with lots of crunchiness as well as vitamin C and B6!

- Prep Time: 20 minutes
- Cook Time: 90 minutes
- Total Time: 110 minutes
- Serving: 2-4

Ingredients

- 2 zucchinis, sliced thin
- 1 tablespoon extra virgin olive oil
- Salt, to taste
- ¼ teaspoon cumin powder (optional)

Instructions

1- Slice zucchinis lengthwise and thin by a slicer.

2- Take out the moisture from zucchinis using clean paper towels. Hold and press down paper towels on zucchinis.
3- Preheat the over to 250 °F.
4- Spray olive oil on parchment papers and then, place zucchinis on them.
5- Spray or pour olive oil on top of zucchinis as well. Sprinkle salt, and cumin powder (optional).
6- Bake zucchinis for about 80-90 minutes until golden.
7- Remove from the oven. Dry zucchinis with a paper towel. Enjoy!

Cooking Tips:

- You can also fry zucchinis in a large pan by extra virgin olive oil over low heat or microwave it. For more crispiness, you may need to broil fried zucchinis.

Nutrition Facts
Servings: 2

Amount per serving	
Calories	**95**
	% Daily Value*
Total Fat 7.4g	10%
Saturated Fat 1.1g	5%
Cholesterol 0mg	0%
Sodium 20mg	1%
Total Carbohydrate 7.2g	3%
Dietary Fiber 2.3g	8%
Total Sugars 3.6g	
Protein 2.5g	
Vitamin D 0mcg	0%
Calcium 32mg	2%
Iron 1mg	5%
Potassium 526mg	11%

Healthy Potato Chips

Crunchy and healthy potato chips can be a tasty snack for IBD patients as they can be made with no oil, and as the snack is fat-free.

- Prep Time: 10 minutes
- Cook Time: 10 minutes
- Total Time: 20 minutes
- Serving: 2

Ingredients

- 2 medium potatoes, skin removed
- ½ teaspoon onion powder (optional)
- Salt, to taste

Instructions

1. Wash potatoes and then, peel-off the skins.
2. Slice potatoes into chips using a very thin slicer.
3. Add salt, and onion powder (optional).
4. Spread all chips on a parchment paper sheet.
5. Put in the microwave until golden brown. Enjoy!

Cooking Tips:

- Potato chips perfectly match with any avocado snack.

Nutrition Facts
Servings: 2

Amount per serving	
Calories	**151**
	% Daily Value*
Total Fat 0.2g	0%
Saturated Fat 0.1g	0%
Cholesterol 0mg	0%
Sodium 13mg	1%
Total Carbohydrate 34.5g	13%
Dietary Fiber 5.2g	19%
Total Sugars 2.8g	
Protein 3.8g	
Vitamin D 0mcg	0%
Calcium 22mg	2%
Iron 1mg	6%
Potassium 880mg	19%

DRINKS

RECOMMENDED HOT BEVERAGES

Recommended hot beverages for IBD patients are:

- Decaffeinated coffee: use decaffeinated coffee instead of caffeinated coffee if you are experiencing a flare-up. When you are in remission, make sure you are taking caffeinated drinks in moderation. It is recommended not to take caffeinated drinks at all if you can.
- Decaffeinated black tea: if you would like to have earl gray, English breakfast, or any types of black tea, it is better to drink decaffeinated kinds, especially if you are experiencing a flare-up. If you are in remission, take caffeinated black tea in moderation. As cinnamon has anti-inflammatory properties, it is a great idea to pour a little bit of cinnamon powder in your black tea.
- Peppermint Tea: this herbal tea is an excellent choice for IBD patients as it has properties that can soothe your digestive tract inflammation. Studies show that peppermint oil can help spasms and cramping in patients with gastrointestinal issues.
- Green Tea: is another excellent choice for IBD patients. It includes polyphenol antioxidants such as epigallocatechin gallate (EGCG), a type of catechin that protects cells from damages and can reduce inflammation that can help chronic conditions. It can also help inhibit bacterial growth, which lowers the risks of getting infections. Moreover, green tea contains less caffeine than regular coffee. However, it could give you a similar mood.
- Ziziphora/Oregano/Thyme Tea: This herbal tea is recommended for people with IBD. Ziziphora is the

name of a mountain plant from the Lamiaceae group, similar to Thyme. It has flavonoids with anti-inflammatory properties. Oregano contains great antioxidants such as Carvacrol and Thymol that can reduce the risk of virus activities. Studies have shown excellent anti-inflammatory properties of oregano. Thyme tea is also great for people with IBD. It has antioxidants and antimicrobial properties with valuable sources of Iron. Thyme can also be used in foods as a great seasoning. You can pour one tablespoon of Ziziphora or Oregano or Thyme in a cup of boiling water and enjoy drinking this fantastic tea after 8-10 minutes.

- <u>Turmeric and Ginger Tea:</u> both turmeric and ginger are fantastic for people living with IBD. Turmeric and Ginger have been used widely in ancient medicine. They use turmeric and ginger as medicines and for better digestion. Turmeric is high in antioxidants that can protect your cells from damaging and reduces the risks of getting infections. Curcumin in turmeric is a great anti-inflammatory ingredient. Ginger also has strong anti-inflammatory properties that can help reduce inflammation in the GI tract.
    - For making a great tea, add ½ teaspoon of ground turmeric and ½ teaspoon of freshly grated ginger in 2 cups of boiling water and enjoy your drink after 12-15 minutes. You can add 1-teaspoon honey or maple syrup to your tea if you can tolerate it. On of the delicious hot beverages you can make with Turmeric and Ginger is called Golden Milk.
    - Golden Milk: mix ½ cup of unsweetened almond milk or lactose-free cow milk, one teaspoon turmeric, ½ teaspoon of freshly

grated ginger, ½ teaspoon of cinnamon powder, and one teaspoon of honey or maple syrup (optional: if you can tolerate) in a small pot and boil. After boiling, simmer for 5 minutes until flavors over low heat.

- Ginger-Mint Tea: you can benefit from both ginger and mint properties by making this great tea. Mint has menthol, which helps reduce inflammation in the gut.

  Boil 10-15 mint leaves with one tablespoon of lemon juice and ½ teaspoon of freshly grated ginger and 2 cups of water in a small pot. Remove from heat, wait for three more minutes and add one tablespoon honey or maple syrup (optional: if you can tolerate) for sweetness if you want.

- Slippery Elm Tea: recent studies showed that slippery elm bark could soothe the stomach and intestinal linings and reducing inflammation and is an excellent drink for people with IBD. Pour one tablespoon of slippery elm in a cup of boiling water and enjoy drinking after 10 minutes.

- Calendula Tea: this tea is known for helping people with peptic ulcers, reflux, and IBD. It can soothe gut inflammation and irritation as it has anti-inflammatory and wound-healing properties. Pour 1 tablespoon of dried calendula in a cup of boiling water and enjoy drinking after 10-12 minutes.

- Milk?: Generally speaking, IBD patients can use low-fat milk if they are in remission and not lactose-intolerant. You can serve milk, hot or cold.
  - Some researchers recommend not to use regular cow milk or any nut/wild rice milk

when you are in a flare-up as milk is hard to be digested.
- If you are in remission and not lactose-intolerant, it is recommended to consume low-fat cow milk, unsweetened almond milk, or rice milk. You can also use soy milk during remissions, but make sure you are using a Non-GMO type. Always check your intolerance level.
- Some patients are lactose-intolerant due to IBD. These patients can use low-fat, lactose-free cow milk, unsweetened almond milk, Non-GMO soy milk, and/or rice milk when they are in remission.

Recommended Cold Beverages

Recommended cold beverages for IBD patients are as below:

- <u>Water:</u> The best drink for IBD patients is water. Try drinking at least 8-10 glasses of water each day, especially if you are experiencing a flare-up, which helps reduce your inflammation and relieve your diarrhea. Try not to use carbonated water if you have IBD.
  - Some patients experienced better feelings of consuming alkaline water with 9.5 pH. Alkaline water is water with a pH of more than 7 (normal). As it has a higher pH than regular water, some claim that it can balance body pH level. Most soda drinks in the market have acidic properties (pH smaller than 7). Ionized alkaline water can increase hydration as ionization may reduce the size of

molecular clusters of water. Some experts also claimed that as active oxygen in water is a free radical, it might damage healthy tissues. Alkaline water may neutralize active oxygen and avoid those damaging healthy tissues.

- <u>Do not drink</u> soda, carbonated beverages, and caffeinated beverages if you have IBD. These drinks may cause you diarrhea and bloating, which can be active or severe your symptoms.
- <u>Gatorade/Powerade:</u> is a fantastic electrolyte drink for IBD patients if they are in remission. It can help to relieve diarrhea, and it contains useful minerals such as sodium, potassium, and vitamins such as B3, B6, and B12.
  - When you are in flare-up periods, try your electrolyte recipe: First glass: mix one cup of water with ½ teaspoon of sugar or honey and a pinch of salt. Second glass: mix one cup of boiled water with ¼ teaspoon of baking soda. When in hydration, drink half of the first glass and then half of the second glass. Drink more from glasses, respectively, if you are still thirsty.
- <u>Fruit Juices:</u> Fruit juices are excellent sources of vitamins for IBD patients. Juicing is essential for IBD patients, as many of them cannot digest fibers in foods and fruits easily. Hence, they can boost their nutrient intake by juicing. However, people with IBD need to consume specific fruits with specific instructions:
  - Do not use juices with the pulp.

- It is recommended not to add sugar or any artificial sweeteners to juices. If you can tolerate honey, maple syrup, or stevia, you can add them to your juice.
- Make sure peeling off fruit skins when you are juicing them.
- It is recommended to consume peeled and poached fruits/ fruit juices when you are experiencing a severe flare-up.
- The best fruit juice that can be consumed in moderation by IBD patients are:

    Aloe Vera, Papaya, Honeydew Melon, Banana, Carrot, Cantaloupe, Squash, Pumpkin, Cucumber (peeled)
- You may want to try other fruit juices (skin removed) such as apple, peach, mango or pear when you are in remission. You may also juice vegetables such as celery and spinach during your remission period. Always start consuming less and check your tolerance level.
- Many experts recommend not to use fruits with small seeds such as blueberries and strawberries.
- Many IBD patients can't tolerate tomato juice. Try not to consume it, especially if you are in a flare-up.

It is better to purchase organic fruits and always correctly wash fruits first, even if you know that you want to remove their skin.

Chapter 6. Bi-weekly Cooking Plan

This chapter provides you with an example of a biweekly meal plan for remission periods. It can give you an idea of how to create your biweekly plans for remission and flare-up periods.

Here are some of the essential tips you need to remember when you want to make your meal plan for remission periods:

Cooking Plan for Remission Periods:

- Try varieties of foods, but always eat and drink healthy foods.
- If you are lactose-intolerant, try alternative products explained in this book.
- If you are gluten-intolerant, try alternative products explained in this book.
- When you are in remission, it does not mean that you can eat everything. There are still some triggering foods to avoid as they can wake up flares. Always make your meal plan based on your health conditions and non-triggering foods that can be well-tolerated by you.
- If you are sensitive to seafood, you can substitute seafood with other foods with healthy fat and protein sources. Many non-seafood cooking recipes provided for you in this book.
- Remember that it is recommended to eat six portions a day instead of 3 portions. Hence, you can have breakfast, snack (between breakfast and lunch), lunch, snack (between lunch and dinner), dinner, and

snack (between dinner and your sleep time). You can use appetizers, snacks, desserts, and snack recipes in this book for snack portions. Alternatively, you can have soups or salads as before-lunch or before-dinner snacks.

Here is an example of a biweekly meal plan for remission Periods:

Week-1:	Week-2:
Monday	**Monday**
Breakfast: Avocado Egg Breakfast Toast **Snack-1:** Zucchini Chips **Lunch:** Chicken Kebab (From Last Night) **Snack-2:** Banana Milkshake **Dinner:** Grilled Honey Salmon and/or Carrot Potato Soup **Snack-3:** Diced Fruits **Drinks:** Coffee, Peppermint Tea	**Breakfast:** Egg Tacos with Avocado **Snack-1:** Gluten-Free Rice Crackers **Lunch:** Chicken Stroganoff (From Last Night) **Snack-2:** Cooler Drink or Almond Butter Toast **Dinner:** Lemon Steamed Halibut with White Rice **Snack-3:** Apple Ginger Sundae **Drinks:** Earl Gray Tea, Green Tea
Tuesday	**Tuesday**
Breakfast: Almond Butter Banana Sandwich **Snack-1:** Gluten-Free Ginger Biscuit **Lunch:** Grilled Honey Salmon and/or Carrot Potato Soup **Snack-2:** Avocado Smoothie **Dinner:** Potato Cutlet with Stracciatella Soup **Snack-3:** Applesauce **Drinks:** Decaffeinated Black Tea, Green Tea	**Breakfast:** Fruit Salad with Almond Milk **Snack-1:** Avocado Dip **Lunch:** Lemon Steamed Halibut with White Rice **Snack-2:** Banana Cinnamon Smoothie **Dinner:** Classic Tuna Pasta Salad or Butternut Squash Soup **Snack-3:** Pomegranate Angelica Drink **Drinks:** Decaffeinated Coffee, Peppermint Tea
Wednesday	**Wednesday**
Breakfast: Apple Cinnamon Oatmeal **Snack-1:** Tofu Toast **Lunch:** Potato Cutlet with Stracciatella Soup **Snack-2:** Cantaloupe Smoothie **Dinner:** Balsamic Peach Pork **Snack-3:** Poached Fruit Compote **Drinks:** Decaffeinated Coffee, Peppermint Tea	**Breakfast:** Oatmeal **Snack-1:** Guacamole-Like Snack **Lunch:** Classic Tuna Pasta Salad or Butternut Squash Soup **Snack-2:** Banana Milkshake **Dinner:** Olivier/Potato Salad with Pumpkin Soup **Snack-3:** Cantaloupe Mix Smoothie **Drinks:** Coffee, Oregano Tea
Thursday	**Thursday**
Breakfast: Gluten-Free Fluffy Pancakes **Snack-1:** Cheese Sticks **Lunch:** Balsamic Peach Pork **Snack-2:** Peach Mango Banana Smoothie **Dinner:** Thunfisch Pizza and/or Butternut Squash Soup **Snack-3:** Gluten-Free Apple Pie **Drinks:** Black Tea with Cinnamon, Ginger Mint Tea	**Breakfast:** Baked Apple **Snack-1:** Avocado Cheese Bagel **Lunch:** Olivier/Potato Salad with Pumpkin Soup **Snack-2:** Baba Ghanoush **Dinner:** Grilled Beef Kebab with White Rice **Snack-3:** Carrot Juice with Mango Ice Cream **Drinks:** Decaffeinated Earl Grey Tea, Ginger Mint Tea
Friday	**Friday**
Breakfast: Two Poached Eggs with Toasts **Snack-1:** Almond Butter Sandwich **Lunch:** Thunfisch Pizza and/or Butternut Squash Soup **Snack-2:** Banana Cinnamon Smoothie	**Breakfast:** Almond Butter Honey Banana Toast **Snack-1:** Applesauce **Lunch:** Grilled Beef Kebab with White Rice **Snack-2:** Carrot Avocado Salad

Dinner: Chicken Zucchini Stew with Chicken Broth **Snack-3:** Diced Fruits such as Papaya **Drinks:** Decaffeinated Coffee, Ziziphora Tea	**Dinner:** Chicken Pizza **Snack-3:** Warm Apple Crumble **Drinks:** Decaffeinated Coffee, Green Tea
Saturday	Saturday
Breakfast: Avocado Cheese Bagel **Snack-1:** Poached Fruits with Plain Yogurt **Lunch:** Chicken Zucchini Stew with Chicken Broth **Snack-2:** Butter Lettuce Salad **Dinner:** Hungarian Goulash with Bone Broth **Snack-3:** Lemon Sorbet or a Fruit Juice **Drinks:** Coffee, Turmeric Ginger Tea	**Breakfast:** Egg Salmon Avocado **Snack-1:** Tofu Toast **Lunch:** Chicken Pizza **Snack-2:** Applesauce Avocado Smoothie **Dinner:** Chicken & Shrimp Teriyaki with Rice Noodles **Snack-3:** Rice Pudding **Drinks:** Coffee, Turmeric Ginger Tea
Sunday	Sunday
Breakfast: Smoothie Bowl with Almond Milk **Snack-1:** Gluten-Free Rice Crackers **Lunch:** Hungarian Goulash with Bone Broth **Snack-2:** Hummus **Dinner:** Chicken Stroganoff **Snack-3:** Avocado Peach Popsicle **Drinks:** Decaffeinated Coffee, Slippery Elm Tea	**Breakfast:** Zucchini Bread Oatmeal **Snack-1:** Gluten-Free Ginger Biscuit **Lunch:** Chicken & Shrimp Teriyaki with Rice Noodles **Snack-2:** Apple Pear Salad **Dinner:** Ginger Sticky Pork **Snack-3:** Pear Cake Sundae **Drinks:** Decaffeinated Black Tea, Calendula Tea

Here are some of the critical points you need to remember when you want to make your meal plan for flare-up periods:

COOKING PLAN FOR FLARE-UP PERIODS

- You have to limit yourself to non-triggering healthy food recipes.
- It is recommended to avoid consuming lactose and gluten during flares.
- Remember: when you are in a flare, you have to put more non-triggering soups, juices, and broth in your meal plan.
- Always make your meal plan based on your health conditions and non-triggering foods that can be well-tolerated by you.

- During flares, stick to your meal plan and modify it only if you found any intolerable foods/ingredients.
- Put more foods with anti-inflammatory herbs and spices such as turmeric and ginger in your flare-up meal plan.
- Drink safe anti-inflammatory herbal teas such as peppermint and green tea during flare-up periods.
- If you are sensitive to seafood, you can substitute seafood with other foods with healthy fat and protein sources. Many non-seafood cooking recipes provided for you in this book.
- Remember that it is recommended to eat six portions a day instead of three portions. Hence, you can have breakfast, snack (between breakfast and lunch), lunch, snack (between lunch and dinner), dinner, and snack (between dinner and your sleep time). You can use appetizers, snacks, desserts, and snack recipes in this book for snack portions. Alternatively, you can have soups or salads as before-lunch or before-dinner snacks.
- If you have issues in making an effective meal plan for your flare-up periods, ask support from a nutritionist or a dietitian. Here is an example of a biweekly flare-up meal plan:

Week-1:	Week-2:
Monday	**Monday**
Breakfast: Avocado + 2 Poached Eggs **Snack-1:** Zucchini Salad **Lunch:** Chicken Kebab with White Rice (From Last Night) **Snack-2:** Carrot Juice **Dinner:** Boiled Salmon / Carrot Potato Soup **Snack-3:** Diced Non-Triggering Fruits **Drinks:** Decaffeinated Coffee, Peppermint Tea	**Breakfast:** Two Poached Eggs with Avocado **Snack-1:** Avocado Dip **Lunch:** Chicken Noodle Soup (From Last Night) **Snack-2:** Cooler Drink **Dinner:** Lemon Steamed Halibut with White Rice **Snack-3:** Ginger Fruit Sherbet (Sweetened by Stevia) **Drinks:** Decaffeinated Black Tea, Green Tea
Tuesday	**Tuesday**
Breakfast: Smooth Almond Butter Banana Sandwich **Snack-1:** Gluten-Free Ginger Biscuit or Rice Crackers **Lunch:** Boiled Salmon / Carrot Potato Soup **Snack-2:** Cantaloupe Juice **Dinner:** Turkey Pot Pie Soup **Snack-3:** Applesauce **Drinks:** Decaffeinated Black Tea, Green Tea	**Breakfast:** Fruit Salad **Snack-1:** Oatmeal (if tolerable) or Firm Tofu **Lunch:** Lemon Steamed Halibut with White Rice **Snack-2:** Carrot Juice **Dinner:** Classic Tuna Pasta Salad + One Bone Broth Cup **Snack-3:** Pomegranate Angelica Drink **Drinks:** Decaffeinated Coffee, Peppermint Tea
Wednesday	**Wednesday**
Breakfast: Oatmeal (if tolerable) or Safe Fruit Bowl **Snack-1:** Firm Tofu Toast **Lunch:** Turkey Pot Pie Soup **Snack-2:** Honeydew Melon Juice **Dinner:** Bone Broth + Carrot Avocado Salad **Snack-3:** Poached Fruit Compote (e.g., Peeled Apple) **Drinks:** Green Tea, Peppermint Tea	**Breakfast:** Oatmeal (if tolerable) or a Safe Fruit Bowl **Snack-1:** Guacamole-Like Snack **Lunch:** Classic Tuna Pasta Salad + One Bone Broth Cup **Snack-2:** Diced Banana **Dinner:** Potato Salad + Pumpkin Soup **Snack-3:** Cantaloupe Juice **Drinks:** Green Tea, Peppermint Tea
Thursday	**Thursday**
Breakfast: Two Poached Eggs with Toasts **Snack-1:** Diced Fruits **Lunch:** Bone Broth + Carrot Avocado Salad **Snack-2:** Applesauce Avocado Smoothie (Lactose-Free) **Dinner:** Butternut Squash Soup **Snack-3:** Cantaloupe or Watermelon Juice **Drinks:** Decaffeinated Black Tea, Ginger Mint Tea	**Breakfast:** Baked Apple **Snack-1:** Smooth Almond Butter Sandwich **Lunch:** Potato Salad + Pumpkin Soup **Snack-2:** Poached Egg Avocado White Pita **Dinner:** Turkey Zucchini Noodles **Snack-3:** Carrot Juice **Drinks:** Decaffeinated Earl Grey Tea, Ginger Mint Tea
Friday	**Friday**

Breakfast: Avocado + Gluten-Free Bagel **Snack-1:** Almond Butter Sandwich **Lunch:** Butternut Squash Soup **Snack-2:** Applesauce **Dinner:** Chicken Zucchini Stew with Chicken Broth **Snack-3:** Diced Fruits such as Papaya **Drinks:** Decaffeinated Coffee, Peppermint Tea	**Breakfast:** Almond Butter Honey Banana Toast **Snack-1:** Applesauce **Lunch:** Turkey Zucchini Noodles **Snack-2:** Carrot Avocado Salad **Dinner:** Butternut Squash Soup **Snack-3:** Lemon Sorbet **Drinks:** Peppermint Tea, Green Tea
Saturday	**Saturday**
Breakfast: Smooth Almond Butter Banana Sandwich **Snack-1:** Poached Fruits (Unsweetened or with Stevia) **Lunch:** Chicken Zucchini Stew with Chicken Broth **Snack-2:** Ginger Cool Drink **Dinner:** Bone Broth and Mashed Potato with No Milk **Snack-3:** Lemon Sorbet **Drinks:** Turmeric Ginger Tea, Turmeric Ginger Tea	**Breakfast:** 2 Poached Eggs with Avocado **Snack-1:** Firm Tofu Toast **Lunch:** Butternut Squash Soup **Snack-2:** Papaya Dices **Dinner:** Lemon Shrimp with White Rice **Snack-3:** Rice Pudding (Unsweetened or by Stevia) **Drinks:** Decaffeinated Coffee, Turmeric Ginger Tea
Sunday	**Sunday**
Breakfast: Smoothie Bowl with Almond Milk **Snack-1:** Gluten-Free Rice Crackers or Applesauce **Lunch:** Bone Broth and Mashed Potato with No Milk **Snack-2:** Guacamole Like Snack **Dinner:** Chicken Noodle Soup **Snack-3:** Popsicle from a Non-triggering Fruit **Drinks:** Decaffeinated Coffee, Green Tea	**Breakfast:** Zucchini Bread Oatmeal **Snack-1:** Gluten-Free Ginger Biscuit **Lunch:** Lemon Shrimp with White Rice **Snack-2:** Apple Pear Salad **Dinner:** Stracciatella Soup + Zucchini Salad **Snack-3:** Popsicle from a Non-triggering Fruit **Drinks:** Decaffeinated Black Tea, Peppermint Tea

BIWEEKLY COOKING PLAN FOR IBD PATIENTS – BLANK

This section gives you two free blank meal plan tables that can be filled by you if you want to create your biweekly plans for remission and flare-up periods.

Biweekly Meal Plan for Remission Periods	
Week-1:	**Week-2:**
Monday	Monday
Breakfast: Snack-1: Lunch: Snack-2: Dinner: Snack-3: Drinks:	Breakfast: Snack-1: Lunch: Snack-2: Dinner: Snack-3: Drinks:
Tuesday	Tuesday
Breakfast: Snack-1: Lunch: Snack-2: Dinner: Snack-3: Drinks:	Breakfast: Snack-1: Lunch: Snack-2: Dinner: Snack-3: Drinks:
Wednesday	Wednesday
Breakfast: Snack-1: Lunch: Snack-2: Dinner: Snack-3: Drinks:	Breakfast: Snack-1: Lunch: Snack-2: Dinner: Snack-3: Drinks:
Thursday	Thursday
Breakfast: Snack-1: Lunch: Snack-2: Dinner: Snack-3: Drinks:	Breakfast: Snack-1: Lunch: Snack-2: Dinner: Snack-3: Drinks:
Friday	Friday
Breakfast: Snack-1: Lunch: Snack-2: Dinner: Snack-3: Drinks:	Breakfast: Snack-1: Lunch: Snack-2: Dinner: Snack-3: Drinks:
Saturday	Saturday
Breakfast: Snack-1: Lunch: Snack-2: Dinner: Snack-3: Drinks:	Breakfast: Snack-1: Lunch: Snack-2: Dinner: Snack-3: Drinks:
Sunday	Sunday
Breakfast: Snack-1: Lunch: Snack-2: Dinner: Snack-3: Drinks:	Breakfast: Snack-1: Lunch: Snack-2: Dinner: Snack-3: Drinks:

Biweekly Meal Plan for Flare-Up Periods	
Week-1:	**Week-2:**
Monday	Monday
Breakfast: Snack-1: Lunch: Snack-2: Dinner: Snack-3: Drinks:	Breakfast: Snack-1: Lunch: Snack-2: Dinner: Snack-3: Drinks:
Tuesday	Tuesday
Breakfast: Snack-1: Lunch: Snack-2: Dinner: Snack-3: Drinks:	Breakfast: Snack-1: Lunch: Snack-2: Dinner: Snack-3: Drinks:
Wednesday	Wednesday
Breakfast: Snack-1: Lunch: Snack-2: Dinner: Snack-3: Drinks:	Breakfast: Snack-1: Lunch: Snack-2: Dinner: Snack-3: Drinks:
Thursday	Thursday
Breakfast: Snack-1: Lunch: Snack-2: Dinner: Snack-3: Drinks:	Breakfast: Snack-1: Lunch: Snack-2: Dinner: Snack-3: Drinks:
Friday	Friday
Breakfast: Snack-1: Lunch: Snack-2: Dinner: Snack-3: Drinks:	Breakfast: Snack-1: Lunch: Snack-2: Dinner: Snack-3: Drinks:
Saturday	Saturday
Breakfast: Snack-1: Lunch: Snack-2: Dinner: Snack-3: Drinks:	Breakfast: Snack-1: Lunch: Snack-2: Dinner: Snack-3: Drinks:
Sunday	Sunday
Breakfast: Snack-1: Lunch: Snack-2: Dinner: Snack-3: Drinks:	Breakfast: Snack-1: Lunch: Snack-2: Dinner: Snack-3: Drinks:

LAST WORDS...

This book aimed to provide you with useful information about low residue diet healthy nutritional choices, food preparation, how to cook for people who needs to follow a low fiber low residue diet and essential dietary tips you need to follow to effectively manage your gastrointestinal disease. It also guided you through meal planning and how to create biweekly cooking plans.

Comprehensive lists of foods to avoid and foods to each for people who want to follow the low residue diet presented in Chapter 2, and Chapter 3 and 4 suggested essential tips for food preparation and meal planning. You learned more than 120 different cooking recipes presented in Chapter 5 of this book, including cooking tips and low residue diet-related tips.

Chapter 6 presented biweekly cooking plan samples. The blanked biweekly cooking plan tables in this chapter can be used by you to write your own cooking plans. Remember that it is always essential to talk to your doctor about suggested foods or any recommended diets you would like to follow.

Now, you have read and learned almost all the basics about low residue-related diets, food preparation, and meal plans by reading this book. If you would like to know about Inflammatory Bowel Diseases (IBD) called Crohn's disease and Ulcerative Colitis in detail and how to manage them to have a better lifestyle, you can read the following books in the amazon kindle/paperback store written by the same author of this book:

The Comprehensive Guide to Crohn's Disease, All You Need to Know About Crohn's Disease, from Diagnosis to Management & Treatment, by Monet Manbacci, P.h.D., Available in Amazon Kindle and Paperback formats, 2019.

Crohn's Disease Comprehensive Diet Guide and Cookbook, by Monet Manbacci, P.h.D., Available in Amazon Kindle and Paperback formats, 2019.

Ulcerative Colitis Comprehensive Diet Guide and Cookbook, by Monet Manbacci, P.h.D., Available in Amazon Kindle & Paperback Formats, 2020.

Moreover, if you found out that you would like to have a comprehensive journal/diary or a calendar that has been designed explicitly for IBD patients to record all your disease-related history, you may want to take a look at the following book in the amazon store prepared by the same author of this book:

My IBD Management Journal: A Beautiful Journal for Ulcerative Colitis and Crohn's disease Patients (Golden Series), by Monet Manbacci, P.h.D., Available in Amazon Paperback Format, Dec. 2019.

ONE LAST THING…

The author of this book would like to thank you for reading this book and hope the book was helpful to you.

If you found this book useful or learned something from it, It would be much appreciated if you write a short review on the Amazon website.

The success of such books highly depends on your honest reviews. Your reviews can help the author improve the quality of this book in the next revisions. It can help other people to make informed decisions about reading this book as well.

If you have any feedback, comments or questions, feel free to email Monet Manbacci: monetmanbacci@gmail.com

Thanks again for your support!

About The Author

Monet Manbacci, Ph.D., is the author of *"Ulcerative Colitis Comprehensive Diet Guide and Cookbook"*, *"The Comprehensive Guide to Crohn's Disease"*, and *"Ulcerative Colitis Journal"* Books. He is an IBD patient who has a Doctor of Philosophy (Ph.D.) degree in Applied Sciences and has been involved in academic and scientific research for more than 14 years.

Other Books By Healthview Publishers:

Crohn's Disease Comprehensive Diet Guide and Cookbook, by Monet Manbacci, P.h.D., Available in Amazon Kindle & Paperback Formats, 2019.

The Comprehensive Guide to Crohn's Disease, All You Need to Know About Crohn's Disease, from Diagnosis to Management & Treatment, by Monet Manbacci, P.h.D., Available in Amazon Kindle & Paperback Formats, 2019.

Ulcerative Colitis Comprehensive Diet Guide and Cookbook, by Monet Manbacci, P.h.D., Available in Amazon Kindle & Paperback Formats, 2020.

Printed in Great Britain
by Amazon